Dr Rachael Morris-Jones is a Dermatology Consultant working at Kings College Hospital, London, UK. She qualified as a doctor over 20 years ago, and has worked in dermatology for 17 years. She does not have any conflict of interest (apart from a passionate belief in preventing and treating skin disease) or any current links to any pharmaceutical companies. She is an enthusiastic and dedicated Honorary Senior Lecturer working for the GKT School of Medicine, Kings College London. She has written several dermatology textbooks and numerous research papers published in the medical literature.

I would like to dedicate this book to all the patients I have treated in the past 20 years who have challenged and tested me to seek out the truth and always look for evidence-based medical knowledge.

Rachael Jones Morris

DERMATOLOGIST TESTED

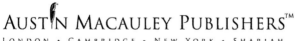
AUSTIN MACAULEY PUBLISHERS™

LONDON • CAMBRIDGE • NEW YORK • SHARJAH

A CIP catalogue record for this title is available from the British Library.

ISBN 9781786930873 (Paperback)
ISBN 9781786930880 (Hardback)
ISBN 9781786930897 (E-Book)
www.austinmacauley.com

First Published (2017)
Austin Macauley Publishers Ltd.
25 Canada Square
Canary Wharf
London
E14 5LQ

I would like to acknowledge all the Dermatology Consultant and Specialist Registrar Dermatology Colleagues that I have worked with at Kings College Hospital, in particular Dr. Elisabeth Higgins who was my mentor for many years and Dr. Sarah Walsh who has always encouraged me to attain my aspirations.

FOREWORD

Skin – the largest organ in the human body; vital to our very existence, keeping our insides in and the outside out. So, what do we really know about our skin, how it stays healthy, what really affects its functioning and appearance and how we heal it when things go wrong? Everywhere we look there are magazine articles, advertisements and health advice columns telling us how we should look after our skin and what leads to skin problems. Equally when we go to the supermarket or the chemist we are bombarded with a bewildering array of products, lotions and potions for every possible skin, hair and nail ailment, but how do we know which ones to choose and if they really work? It can all be quite overwhelming, with lots of mixed messages. How much is fact and how much is fiction or myth? To answer these questions the published evidence has been scrutinised to try to determine the truth on each topic examined.

Most of us are aware that products are usually tested by the company's manufacturing them and therefore this could lead to a bias in the testing process, incomplete reporting of results and only revealing the outcomes that help to support the products use. How do we know we can trust the source of this type of information? What are the measures that say a product works, what is the actual evidence? These studies are frequently published in medical journals, which does enhance their apparent authority on the subject matter: however, we must look at the potential conflicts of interest that may influence the way the papers are written and the way the results are interpreted.

The huge challenge for any of us is unpicking the facts from the fiction particularly when we are faced with often contradictory information from multiple different sources, some of which may be unreliable or even biased. Measuring outcomes in the skin should be relatively easy as the skin is an accessible organ compared to say internal organs such as the brain and lungs. Measures applied to the skin include ultrasound scan to measure skin thickness, tests of elasticity, measurement of how much water is lost from the skin surface (trans-epidermal water loss), and special UV cameras to examine sun damage.

But to see what's really going on in the skin at the cellular level then frequently taking a skin sample or skin biopsy is needed. Taking samples from the skin is quick, simple and relatively risk free; however it usually involves cutting the skin which leaves a small but permanent scar. This can be difficult to justify in an experimental model on volunteers when products are designed to improve the appearance or quality of the skin. To get around this sometimes companies use explants to tests their products on. This is basically some skin cells growing in a petri dish, but how much this relates to 'real life' is difficult to know as the skin is no longer connected to the rest of the body, that has a huge influence on what is going on at the surface.

The other challenge we face is that many doctors themselves feel that their baseline knowledge about the complex workings of the skin and what affects it, may be limited. Which is hardly surprising if we consider that for example in the UK (as in many other countries) many doctors have only a few hours of specific dermatology teaching during their entire five-year medical school training. As doctors, we are encouraged to practice 'evidence-based medicine' and wherever possible this should be our 'gold standard'. However, sometimes this isn't possible if the definitive evidence just isn't available, and then we need to rely on our experience and observations gleaned from many years of clinical practice. We need to remember however that this is anecdotal rather than evidence based medicine.

Nonetheless our generation knows much more than our parents' generation about sun protection and skin cancer and with information freely available on the internet, we are just a click away from advice and guidance. However, we need to try to work out what information is based on actual evidence and what might be based on experience or beliefs, so we can make informed decisions.

Whether we like it or not, many of us live in a society where we can be judged by our outward appearance, so it's hardly surprising that we may feel the pressure to try to achieve 'blemish-free' skin. Superdrug, a large health and beauty retailer in the UK, surveyed its female customers in 2013 and found they spent an average of £250/year on skin care and used an estimated 38 different facial products. Interestingly skincare manufacturers are now increasingly targeting men with male-specific products which are breaking away from the 'traditional three', namely shampoo, deodorant and shaving cream. Many younger men will now use a range of male-specific toiletries including moisturisers, facial cleansers, eye serums and anti-ageing creams. So selling skin care products is big business in many countries.

Dermatologist Tested explores the actual evidence base of our current knowledge about the skin, hair and nails. Questions long held beliefs and myths. Looks for the reality about the effect the outside world has on our skin's function and appearance. And will dig deep to find the truth behind what products and life-style choices can actually help to keep our skin healthy and ease skin conditions.

INTRODUCTION

What/whom are dermatologists?

First of all, what/whom are Dermatologists? And why should you take my word for anything? To answer that question, I just want to give you a quick background on what dermatologists are. In the UK Dermatologists are mainly hospital-based doctors who have undergone general medical training (internal medicine) for between 2-3 years (hospital based training) before sitting and passing a set of post-graduate theory and clinical exams called MRCP (Membership of the Royal College of Physicians). They can then apply for a training position (called a National Training Number, NTN) in dermatology. These training positions are limited (capped by the government) and are highly sought after, dermatology is the second most popular hospital specialty in the UK (after cardiology), so attracts some of the top junior doctors in the country.

The dermatology training then lasts for a minimum of 4 years, with a multitude of competencies that need to achieved before the doctor sits the dermatology specialist exit exam. The doctor is then entered onto the specialist register as a qualified Dermatologist. Quite a few dermatologists then do an extra 1-3 years of dermatology training in a sub-specialist area such as dermatological surgery, paediatric dermatology, allergy etc. and some do laboratory/clinical research (MSc/PhD). So in the UK they are highly trained individuals (minimum training usually 7 years) capable of looking after patients with a multitude of serious skin diseases. In many other countries, such as the USA and parts of Europe dermatologists may do very little general hospital medicine before undertaking specific dermatology training, and they are usually based in clinics/offices rather than in hospitals. Many of them will undertake cosmetic work as well as treating skin disease. So not all dermatologists are the same, but nonetheless they have all undertaken years of specialist training.

So now we understand what a Dermatologist is, let's turn our attention to all the information out there in the public domain about the skin itself, what can go wrong with it and what treatments/products we might use to put things right.

What does 'dermatologically tested' actually mean?

When you pick up any product at the chemist or the supermarket that is designed to be used on the skin, you will often see the message 'dermatologically tested'. This sounds very reassuring, as if the product has been approved by a 'gold standard' for effectiveness and lack of unwanted adverse effects. However, you may be shocked to hear that in fact there is no designated industry-agreed set of tests that needs to be conducted on products for them to claim they are 'dermatologically tested'.

The term conjures up the suggestion in my mind and the public's, that a dedicated medical panel of dermatology specialists have investigated the product's claims, thoroughly tested it, written a report and submitted a conclusion giving the product an official stamp of approval. Unfortunately, this couldn't be further from the truth.

The consumer watchdog body *Which Health* undertook a survey to try to find out what consumers understood by the term 'dermatologically tested'. 25% of those asked thought it meant that the product had been tested on human skin, 32% thought it meant hypoallergenic and 13% that it was 'skin friendly'. In fact, these answers may or may not be true, as we don't know what tests are carried out on the products and we have no idea whether the products passed or failed those tests.

Which Health contacted 10 leading cosmetics companies and asked them to provide evidence to support their claims of 'dermatologically tested' on their products. Of the eight that replied, the information provided didn't give details about the test methods carried out or what result should be achieved. So there is a clear lack of standardisation. As consumers, therefore we are pretty much left in the dark, feeling at best confused and at worst misled about the claims on the packaging.

Tests that are known to be carried out on some products include the 'repeat insult patch test', where usually the product is repeatedly applied to the same area of skin to see if any adverse reaction occurs. Other tests that may be carried out include photopatch testing (product plus ultraviolet light, to check for allergy), photo-toxicity testing (ultraviolet light plus product to test for toxic reactions), cumulative irritant test (any irritation on chronic exposure) and tests for comedogenicity (to check it doesn't block pores). So these tests, if carried out and passed by the products would go some way to increasing our confidence that at least the product is unlikely to do harm.

Wouldn't it be refreshing however, to be told exactly what tests were done on every product and what the results were before we decide to buy? This transparency would be hugely reassuring and would show the company manufacturing the product is committed to quality and safety. In the modern world of the internet where literally any product can be purchased on-line which could be shipped from any country, some evidence to back up the list of the ingredients and safety testing would be welcome.

Some products claim 'dermatologist tested' which is slightly different from dermatologically tested and apparently means that there is an endorsement of the product by one or more dermatologist doctors. However, we don't know if these doctors have any conflicts of interest, such as an association with that brand, have shares in the company, are being paid for their endorsement or are able to access reduced rate products for their patients.

Endorsements by companies or organisations may also feature on products. Often these independent organisations have carried out its own tests on the products and a panel of experts has decided whether to endorse the product or not. The manufacturing/cosmetic company may need to pay for the independent tests to be carried out and occasionally pay an annual 'licence fee' to continue displaying the endorsement.

For example, The British skin foundation (BSF, one of the UK's leading charity supporters of skin disease research) may occasionally be approached to endorse a particular product by a company. The BSF will independently review (at least two consultant dermatologist volunteers, including one expert in the related field) all the research (technical and clinical data supplied by the company) on a particular product to ensure that it is not actually detrimental to skin health.

Interestingly and importantly endorsement by any organisation does not usually mean there is recognition of the product's efficacy or that the product is a market leader. But nonetheless, such endorsements will inevitably give a greater 'weighting' to a product than the one sitting next to it on the shelf without an independent endorsement. There is a fine line to tread for these organisations, endeavouring to remain truly independent and at the same time being linked to particular products.

Products manufactured in the beauty and cosmetics industry may sometimes have scientifically sounding names and ingredients, such as rejuvenating serums, anti-oxidants, microbeads and active enzymes. The company will have ensured the product has undergone some sort of testing that leads to the claim of 'clinically proven'. But what does this actually mean in reality?

'Proven' to most people (including scientists) implies there must have been rigorous research undertaken (such as double-blind, placebo controlled trials) to ensure the products are as efficacious as they claim to be. To date, however, sadly it is often unclear what research has been undertaken on some beauty products whose effectiveness is apparently 'clinically proven'. Scientific work of some sort, however, has usually been carried out, but this is frequently conducted by scientists working for the companies themselves and therefore, some argue, they may have a 'conflict of interest'. If such research is accepted into a *peer reviewed journal* then usually it is of good quality and the findings are in keeping with the conclusions. But not all research makes it into these prestigious journals (the research data may be rejected after scrutiny from independent experts) and some is actually never published.

Most clinical researchers when publishing scientific results refer to 'statistical significance' (related to a p:value, that indicates how likely or not the results could have occurred by chance, the smaller the p:value the more likely the results are significant), rather than reporting that the effects are 'proven'. This is obviously a scientific convention, but it's a standard globally recognised if you really want to prove that something is effective. The most robust studies are placebo controlled (a placebo is a 'fake medicine' such as a 'sugar pill' or just the 'vehicle' that the ingredients are made up in when testing topical treatments (anything directly applied to the skin). This placebo controlled mode of research means that whatever is being investigated is compared to placebo (which usually has a positive effect of its own), so that the active medicine's real worth can be demonstrated.

The challenge for the scientists testing beauty products is finding something tangible that they can measure. For example, taking skin biopsies after a product has been used to show the effects at the cellular level is not normally feasible in human volunteers, but may be carried out on skin explants (skin growing in a petri dish in the lab). So frequently what is reported in human testing is less scientific, such as satisfaction levels of those using the products, which in itself is encouraging, but not really proof of efficacy.

So, what *Dermatologist Tested* endeavours to do, is to look at all the real evidence that is in the published medical literature (mainly peer review journals) to try to see what grounds we actually have for the knowledge base we possess on our skin/hair and nails. Sometimes, with the best will in the world to do that, the evidence just isn't there, and more studies are needed. But where there is evidence, it has been evaluated to guide you through the truths and myths about our skin.

UK Dermatologists at a glance

- They are doctors who have trained and work mainly in hospitals
- Training is in general medicine for 2-3 years and then at least 4 years as a specialist
- Dermatologists have MRCP and CCT in Dermatology
- Dermatologists can subspecialise in skin surgery, paediatrics, allergy, genital disease, photobiology, severe drug reactions, infections and malignancies of the skin etc.
- Most Dermatologists in the UK work in the NHS and the majority do not undertake private practice.

Top tips on looking for the facts/evidence:

- Go to www.ncbi.nlm.nih.gov/**pubmed** then type in the search box the topic you are interested in. A list of relevant published articles will be displayed.

- Look at the British Association of Dermatologists website. This is an excellent source of information concerning multiple skin conditions.

- Go to www.**dermnetnz.org** this is a website written by dermatologists in New Zealand and is an excellent resource. It has great information that is easy to understand and is up to date and factual. Alternatively, if you want to look up a particular skin condition, then type the name of it into a search engine and then type NZ after it (for example eczema nz, melanoma nz), then you will be taken to the dermnetnz.org webpage concerning that condition.

- Cochrane reviews are massive studies conducted by experts who look at all the published medical literature about a certain topic: they grade the studies and then analyse all the findings to draw conclusions and are highly regarded. National Institute for Health and Care Excellence (NICE) is an outstanding organisation based in the UK, responsible for setting up panels of experts to look at medical treatments. They determine whether they are safe and cost-effective, and their evidence guides (NICE Guidelines) what medical practitioners can do.

- Good studies are generally large (often hundreds or thousands of participants), double blinded (neither participants or researchers know which treatment/product has been taken/used, until the final analysis), placebo controlled (compared to fake medicine/product), and published in a peer reviewed journal (independent experts have examined all the data and deemed it reliable).

- When examining research papers look at the conflicts of interests listed for each author so that you can take into account any possible role that may play in the conclusions of the study.

CHAPTER 1

Effects of the Sun on our Body and our Skin

What effects does the sun really have on our general health and on our skin? Is it more beneficial than harmful? If we avoid the sun, then aren't we likely to become vitamin D deficient?

The sun provides energy for all life on earth and has been revered for thousands of years. There is something deeply pleasurable about the feeling of warm sunshine on our skin. Many of us experience an intense sense of wellbeing and lifted spirits when we are out in the sun. So how can something essential to the very existence of life on earth also potentially take life away?

There is mounting evidence from published studies and organisations such as Cancer Research UK and the American Cancer Society that over-exposure to intense sunlight can be harmful to the skin and can even cause death from skin cancer. The World Health Organisation has classified both the ultraviolet (UV) spectrum and artificial UV devices as carcinogenic to humans.

However, we also know that UV radiation (UVR) helps us to make vitamin D in our skin, a substance that is essential for healthy bones and teeth. There is a growing body of research papers suggesting deficiency in vitamin D can leave us vulnerable to multiple sclerosis, Type I diabetes and various types of cancer. So what's the truth about the sun and our health?

Scientific and public opinions are divided. Some people feel that the sun is essentially safe and that they should try to get as much exposure to it as possible. They will travel to sunny places on holiday and sit out all day trying to maximise their exposure by 'bathing' in it. Others see the sun as something powerful and potentially dangerous and will try to avoid it as much as possible. These people stay covered up and stay indoors when it's intensely sunny and encourage others to do the same. So what are we supposed to believe and where does the truth really lie?

Let's firstly take a look at the beneficial effects of the sun on our health and general sense of wellbeing. We are exposed to solar radiation in a regular 24-hour cycle that varies in the number of sunlight hours and intensity with the season. Studies from the University of Alaska have shown that lack of sunlight in the winter months can lead to depression, lethargy, incoherent thinking, craving for carbohydrates and unsociability. Increased sunlight exposure has been linked to increased energy levels and improved mood. Some individuals experience so-called 'seasonal affective disorder' (SAD) which manifests as symptoms of depression that vary with the season. SAD is thought to be linked to shortening daylight hours in the autumn and winter months. So how can sunlight affect our brain? The exact mechanism is unclear but we think that sunlight affects a part of the brain called the hypothalamus, which is responsible for sleep, appetite and mood.

The hypothalamus is considered to be the link between the endocrine and the neurological systems and is responsible for maintaining a balance called 'homeostasis' in the body. Homeostasis helps to control temperature, blood pressure, fluid balance, appetite/thirst, sleep patterns and the release of certain hormones. So UVR or a lack of it can actually affect a significant number of internal processes in the body by affecting the hypothalamus. Sunlight enters the eyes and is passed to the pigmented membrane at the back of our eyes called the retina, which absorbs the light and converts it into nerve messages which pass to the hypothalamus.

The hypothalamus helps to control our internal biological clock called our circadian rhythm. The word 'circa' comes from the Latin to mean around or approximately and 'dia' day. The circadian rhythm is an in-built system that can be affected by external stimuli such as sunlight hours and artificial sources of light. Modern lifestyles often have artificially extended daylight hours which can disrupt our circadian rhythm. It is thought that about 10% of our genes oscillate with our biological 24-hour clock. Many of these genes are responsible for the normal cell cycle, metabolic pathways and repair of damaged DNA.

Therefore in theory, disruption to our natural circadian rhythm may have adverse effects including an increased risk of internal cancers. Sunlight is the main regulator of the circadian rhythm and as a result affects the expression (functioning) of some genes. Artificial light sources can also affect the circadian rhythm, although to a lesser extent. Recent studies have shown that reading from a hand held backlighted device rather than a paper book just before bed delays the onset of sleep by increasing our melatonin levels. Interestingly, melatonin, as well as keeping us awake for longer has a protective role in our skin against damage from UVB and has a powerful anti-oxidant effect. Over the last decade abnormally low levels of melatonin have been shown to be associated with breast, prostate and lung cancer.

So the daily changing rhythm of light-dark periods in humans becomes chemically imprinted on our brains and this affects our sleep patterns, hormone levels and our ability to repair damaged DNA. With this knowledge in mind, spacecraft environments have been adjusted to mimic these naturally occurring light-dark cycles so as to maintain health and wellbeing of the astronauts.

Research carried out on night shift workers in factories has shown a disturbance of these natural rhythms leading to fatigue, low mood, a reduced ability to concentrate and make sound decisions. Many workers in our ever-evolving 24-hour society have a rotating shift pattern: for example emergency medical staff and airline pilots. These rotating shifts have an even more disruptive effect than permanent or long stretches of fixed nights, leading to poor sleep patterns, increased cardiovascular disease, higher perceived stress levels, social isolation and higher divorce rates. So lack of light and disturbed light-dark patterns can adversely affect our health.

People suffering from SAD are usually prescribed electric lamps that simulate the sun leading to correction of their symptoms. In certain circumstances, artificial light sources can be used to substitute for sunlight in resetting the biological clock with associated health benefits.

What about other beneficial effects of the sun? Most of us know that vitamin D is made in the skin when it's exposed to sunlight. Vitamin D is essential to healthy mineralisation of bones, immune responses and even DNA repair mechanisms. With our increasingly indoor lifestyles, sunscreen use and often poor diets many of us are vitamin D deficient. Vitamin D can be absorbed from our diet and synthesized by our skin when exposed to sunlight. But can vitamin D be made in our skin using artificial light sources or do we need actual solar radiation?

Well, an interesting study looking at severely vitamin D deficient patients with cystic fibrosis and short bowel syndrome (these individuals are unable to absorb vitamin D from their gut) was able to show that these patients were able to increase their vitamin D levels in the winter using an artificial light source which mimics sunlight. The patients were initially exposed to 6 minutes of light twice a week for 8 weeks in a light cabinet (similar to a sunbed) and later in a sitting position with only their lower back exposed to a sunlamp placed about 15cm away for 5-10 minutes 5 times per week for 8 weeks. Vitamin D levels increased in all the patients using each method. Leading them to conclude that solar simulated light can increase vitamin D metabolism in the skin.

However some recent studies have shown that not all people respond in the same way and that the vitamin D levels may taper off despite ongoing sunlamp exposure. So at the moment using artificial light sources to try to increase or maintain vitamin D levels may help some individuals but is not recommended for the general public. So for most of us, we would be more certain of increasing our vitamin D levels by taking dietary supplements rather than by exposing ourselves to artificial solar simulators.

So we know that sunlight is beneficial at increasing our vitamin D levels, but how much skin do you need to expose and how much sunlight do you need to synthesize sufficient levels of vitamin D? Do you need to lie out in the sun scantily clad or does walking down the road with just face and hands exposed offer sufficient skin surface to make adequate amounts of vitamin D?

Firstly, we need to decide what level of vitamin D in our blood is needed for healthy body functioning. A simple enough question but the answer is less straightforward as vitamin D has multiple roles in the body and each person has different requirements. However, experts have concluded that levels of vitamin D above 35-40ng/ml (90-100nmol/L) are needed for healthy body functioning (bone and muscle strength, dental health) and may help in prevention of some diseases that may be associated with low levels of vitamin D (such as colorectal cancer and multiple sclerosis). Other authors however have suggested that a higher level of 60ng/ml is desirable. The debate continues, but at least we have a rough guide level of vitamin D to aim for.

Doctors can request a blood test to determine if their patients have sufficient vitamin D levels. The test measures the serum level of 25-OH vitamin D. Deficiency is usually defined as levels below 20ng/ml and insufficiency as levels between 21-35ng/ml. Oral vitamin D supplements can be taken by those with vitamin D deficiency or insufficiency to increase their levels. It is estimated that in the context of deficiency a dose of 800-1000 international units (IU) of vitamin D (equivalent to 20-25mcg) daily would be required for over 3 months to reach normal levels and then supplements would need to continue (at about 400IU or 10mcg daily) to maintain normal vitamin D levels.

How much sun would we need on our skin to ensure sufficient levels of vitamin D? As you might expect the answer is, it depends - on the intensity of the sunlight, cloud cover and your skin tone. Scientists in Norway at the Institute for Air Research have devised a calculator that will take all these factors into account and then estimate how many minutes of sun exposure you will need to produce 25mcg (1000IU) of vitamin D. If you want to do your own calculations then you need to enter a bit of data, but don't let that put you off, it's an interesting exercise. You need the latitude and longitude of your location and the altitude in kilometres (you can look this up on the internet), the thickness of the ozone layer (I suggest you just use 'medium' for this), the time of the year and the time of day and finally your skin type (in terms of how fair or dark your skin is).

Below is a table with an example worked out using the Norwegian group's calculator (Webb *et al*). I have selected the location of London, UK. So basically a temperate climate with sunlight that is not usually very intense. I selected 'broken/scattered cloud' for this example (as that is common to have cloud in the UK throughout the year!) and we are assuming only the face, hands and arms are exposed. Time of day was set to midday. The ground selected is 'dry concrete' (reflected sunlight levels are affected by the ground type). The number of hours/minutes shown is the amount of time in the sun required to synthesize 25mcg (1000IU) of vitamin D, if exposed every other day.

Webb, A.R. and O. Engelsen (2006) Calculated Ultraviolet Exposure Levels for a Healthy Vitamin D Status. Photochemistry and Photobiology. 82(6), 1697-1703.

Follow this link to do your own calculation: http://nadir.nilu.no/~olaeng/fastrt/VitD-ez_quartMEDandMED.html

London, UK sunlight minutes needed <u>alternate days</u> to exposed skin (face/hands/arms) to synthesize 25mcg Vitamin D.

Skin type	1st April	1st August	1st December
Pale Caucasian	8 minutes	5 minutes	2 hours 20 mins
Blond Caucasian	11 minutes	6 minutes	3 hours 8 mins
Darker Caucasian	13 minutes	7 minutes	4 hours 16 mins
Mediterranean	20 minutes	11 minutes	>24 hours
Middle Eastern	26 minutes	14 minutes	>24 hours
Black	44 minutes	24 minutes	>24 hours

So as we would expect in the spring and summer we need a lot less time in the sun to synthesize sufficient vitamin D compared to the winter. In fact in the winter in London we would all have a lot of difficulty in making sufficient vitamin D in our skin from the sun.

Luckily in the winter we can usually rely on our vitamin D stores in the body to tide us over until the spring. We can also get additional vitamin D from our diet. Vitamin D is oil soluble which means you need to eat fat to absorb it (bear this in mind if you are on a low-fat diet). Foods naturally high (or artificially fortified) in vitamin D include cod liver oil, oily fish (salmon, sardines, kippers, pilchards, fresh tuna, trout, swordfish, mackerel), mushrooms, cheese, eggs, tofu, fortified cereals, fortified milk, soya and almond milk. Other commonly fortified foods include orange juice, bread, margarine, yoghurt and infant formula.

In India vitamin D deficiency is endemic despite plenty of sunshine. Experts have supposed this was due to cultural practices not facilitating adequate sun exposure. However, an intriguing study conducted in Hawaii in 2007 showed that of the 93 adults tested (mean age 24 years), 51% had a vitamin D level <30ng/ml despite reporting an average of 28 hours of sun exposure per week. So skin exposure to sunlight can't be the whole story, perhaps we don't all synthesize vitamin D effectively from sunlight, or perhaps we don't take enough or absorb sufficient vitamin D from our diets?

In India, to try to combat almost an entire population being vitamin D deficient the government has been looking at trying to fortify staple foods. One widely eaten food called sattu (a protein rich food made of roasted flour, cereals and legumes) has been identified as an ideal candidate for fortification as it is frequently served in schools for children's lunches. So this is a population-based health intervention that should at least replenish vitamin D stores of school children.

We still have a long way to go to ensure globally we are all getting sufficient vitamin D from the sun and our food. Most of us will need a combination of sunshine and vitamin D rich foods to sustain adequate levels and how much of each of these we need will depend on the strength of the sunlight where we live, our skin type, how much of our skin is exposed to the sun, our individual body demands for vitamin D (higher in childhood and pregnancy), how much vitamin D is in our food and how well we are absorbing it from our gut. So there are multiple factors that will vary from person to person.

The heated debate in the medical literature continues unabated, arguing for and against the potential role of vitamin D insufficiency/deficiency in potentially multiple different diseases. One such disease is multiple sclerosis (MS). We have known now for a number of years that MS is more common in temperate climates than tropical climates. The further away from the equator you live, the higher your risk. So lack of sunshine and vitamin D deficiency could be the link. Studies of people who moved to another country during childhood showed that children adopt the risk of developing MS of the country they move to. However, if they moved after the age of 20 years they kept the risk of the country they originally came from. This suggests that the childhood environment may influence the risk of developing MS. Also, a group in Oxford identified a link between vitamin D and a gene known to be associated with MS. They showed that when vitamin D was present the signal from the gene was stronger, and when absent, the signal was weaker. So could increasing vitamin D levels in those suffering from MS help? Sadly, to date there are no studies showing giving vitamin D supplements to MS patients helps to prevent relapses or improve levels of disability, which is obviously disappointing.

So what about the potential harmful effects of the sun? Most of the current concerns relate to damage to the skin and the eyes. Excessive UVR, particularly UVB on the eyes, causes inflammation of the cornea called photokeratitis. Prolonged periods of sun exposure lead to direct injury to the superficial outer layer of the cornea (the epithelium), the lens and the retina. This is more likely to occur when the sun is very intense, such as looking at a solar eclipse or sun highly reflected by snow (so-called 'snow blindness'). Artificial light sources can also cause corneal damage such as welder's arc 'flash burns', tanning beds and halogen lamps. Consequences of excessive UVR on the eye include certain types of cataracts, macular degeneration and photokeratitis.

Protective eyewear is usually all that is required to prevent the eye from such damage. Modern sunglasses are pretty sophisticated, many quality ones can block 99-100% of UVA and UVB. In addition to UV protection some lenses are polarizing which helps to reduce reflected glare from water and snow. Photochromic lenses darken or lighten depending on how much light is available and for extra protection wrap-around or close-fitting sunglasses with wide lenses protect the eyes from every sunlight angle.

The paler your eye colour the more at risk you are from the sun, and this is also true for the skin: the paler your skin the more at risk you are from the harmful effects of intense sunlight. 95% of solar radiation consists of ultraviolet A (UVA) and 5% is ultraviolet B (UVB). UVA is around all year at the same levels and can pass through clouds (UVA has a long wavelength that hits the earth during winter and summer at the same level, if there is sun, then there is UVA). UVB is at its highest levels in the summer months and in the middle of the day (UVB has a short wavelength and therefore they only hit the earth when it's closer to the sun in the summer).

When sunlight hits the surface of our skin UVB penetrates into the top layer (called the epidermis) and UVA penetrates more deeply into the dermis, which sits just below the epidermis. The solar energy is transmitted and scattered into the skin tissue and effects our cells, proteins, collagen, elastic fibres and deoxyribonucleic acid (DNA).

The result of this UVR in the skin is inflammation of the tissues and some level of damage to the DNA (which contains the genetic instructions for cell functioning). Damage to the DNA can cause mutation and disease, including skin cancer. Luckily, we have an inbuilt repair mechanism called nucleotide excision repair (NER) for correcting any damage to our DNA, whatever the cause. NER is a complex process involving at least 30 genes and 4 steps in the correction process. Sunlight is well recognised to cause abnormalities in the DNA and these must be correctly identified and repaired by the NER. So you can imagine, the more UVR the skin is exposed to the more potential DNA damage occurs and the more repairs that will need to take place. Eventually one of these errors could be missed by the NER, leading to an uncorrected DNA mutation that might lead to skin cancer.

It has been estimated that in one day of intense UVR exposure, one million individual DNA errors can be triggered in the skin. Not all of these will cause structural damage to the DNA, but nonetheless the DNA will need to be repaired. So exposing fair skin to very intense sunlight repeatedly might be considered to be a bit like playing Russian roulette, eventually some of the DNA might not be repaired properly and if that cell doesn't undergo apoptosis (programmed cell death), then the abnormality remains in the skin and can lead to the formation of skin cancer.

There are three main types of skin cancer: melanoma, squamous cell carcinoma and basal cell carcinoma. Worldwide there are more new cases of skin cancer every year than the total combined cases of prostate, colon, breast and lung cancer. However, the good news is that the most common form of skin cancer, called basal cell carcinoma, is relatively easy to treat and rarely leads to death. Melanoma, which is the fifth commonest cancer diagnosed in the UK, accounts for less than 2% of skin cancer cases. Melanoma, however, is more harmful than the other types of skin cancer and can lead to death. So, the most common type of skin cancer is the most harmless and the rarest type the most harmful.

A recent survey of >1000 adults carried out in the UK by the British Association of Dermatologists found that 85% were worried about skin cancer. 72% of those surveyed also reported at least one episode of sunburn in the past year. We know that sustaining sunburn doubles our chance of developing skin cancer in the future, and we are more susceptible to sunburn if we have a fair skin tone. Melanoma for example occurs in 1 in 50 white Americans (1 in 18 Australians, 1 in 55 UK citizens), 1 in 200 Hispanics and 1 in 1000 African Americans. Sun protection advice therefore is trying to reduce our individual risk of developing skin cancer, which in the USA affects 1 in 5 adults.

So, avoiding sunburn seems to very important in protecting ourselves from the potentially harmful effects of the sun.

Top tips associated with light/sunlight

- Try to avoid using a backlighted device for reading before going to sleep.

- Try to eat plenty of vitamin D rich foods such as oily fish, eggs, tofu, soya/almond milk.

- Small amounts of UV exposure are usually sufficient for normal levels of vitamin D.

- If you're concerned about your vitamin D level, think about getting it checked.

- If you have low vitamin D take dietary supplements rather than increased UV exposure.

- Wear photo-protective sunglasses in bright sunlight to protect your eyes.

- Try to avoid sunburn (info in chapter 3) to reduce your risk of skin cancer increasing.

CHAPTER 2

What is Skin Tanning?

What happens to our skin as we tan? What are freckles? Are sunbeds really harmful? Is the only safe tan a fake tan?

I am sure in the past you have heard people commenting on someone's appearance being 'pale and sickly' or that they have a 'healthy tan'. In modern society, we have a tendency to associate having a tanned skin with a sign of health and well-being. It could be the assumption that the tanning may be associated with a restful holiday or relaxation/leisure activities. The Victorians looked upon a tan as a sign of someone who worked outdoors as a labourer and the gentry would usually have pale skin, which they protected with a parasol when out in the sun. So, the appeal of a tan certainly does change with the era and the fashion. Also in modern societies, there are cultural differences as to the desirability of being tanned or preserving our natural skin tone.

Tanning occurs hours or days after exposure to sunlight (or indeed artificial lights such as phototherapy/sunbeds) and persists for weeks or even months in some people. Melanin is the brown pigment in our skin and it's made by cells called melanocytes. Whatever our skin tone we all have the same number of melanocytes near the surface of our skin, but their ability to produce melanin pigment varies, such that pale skinned people naturally produce little melanin whereas darker skinned people make more melanin.

When we are out in the sun, granules of melanin pigment close to the skin surface are oxidised by the UV light and turn a darker colour. The melanocytes which are underneath the top layer of the skin become activated and make more melanin granules, which are then passed to the surface cells called keratinocytes. Inside the keratinocytes, the melanin granules are positioned like a brown 'hat' to cover the cell's nucleus which contains the vulnerable DNA. The melanocytes in the skin layer below remain active for about 5-7 days after the sunlight exposure and continue to produce more melanin granules ready for later.

The 'brown hat' in the keratinocytes is the brown colour that we see as a tan, so really tanning is a protection mechanism against UV damage to our cells. Melanocytes in most of us are spread out evenly in our skin, however in some of us the melanocytes are in clumps which appear as freckles. Simple freckles are small brown flat spots that can develop from a very young age as a reaction to the sun in those with red hair and/or a fair skin. Freckles tend to develop on the most vulnerable sites where the skin is thinnest, such as the nose, cheeks, ears and backs of the hands. The keratinocytes which contain the 'brown hat' of melanin make up the top layers of our skin and as the skin undergoes its normal turn-over process and old cells shed, then the tan 'fades'. Freckles however remain, although they can fade a little in the winter months.

The tendency to form freckles in the sun is genetic and is often linked to having red hair. Skin pigment production relates to the activity of the MC1R gene. When MC1R is working well it produces brown pigment (eumelanin) and when it's not working so well it leads to red pigment (pheomelanin) and sometimes freckles.

If we have pale skin (i.e. not many of those superficial melanin granules) then we are more likely to sustain a sunburn than if we have lots of them (a naturally darker tone of skin). In sunburn we are unable to produce a sufficiently protective oxidised layer of melanin granules in the top layer of our skin as soon as the sun shines down on us, and therefore our cells underneath are left vulnerable to the damaging effects of intense UV and can be killed (the dead cells are called 'sunburn cells') or can be damaged so that they mutate but don't die.

We see and feel this damage as red, warm, painful and swollen skin that can sometimes even blister. At this stage, we can try to calm down the affected skin with cooling oily creams, steroid ointments, anti-inflammatory medicines such as ibuprofen or even oral steroid tablets (prednisolone). As areas of sunburn settle 'sunburn freckles' can develop. These are brown flat spots on the skin that look slightly larger and more irregular than simple freckles.

Over time if we expose our skin to more sun than it can naturally take then it may develop multiple 'age spots' or 'liver spots' which often appear on the backs of our hands or on the face. In fact they have nothing to do with the liver or aging, but are a marker of too much sun (solar lentigo) over the years in a person with fair skin. Freckles in themselves are harmless but they are a marker that in a genetically susceptible individual the skin has been exposed to more sun than it was able to handle effectively.

With chronic exposure to the sun day after day or even month after month, fair skin will also react by thickening up, sometimes to three or four times the thickness of sun-protected skin, giving it a somewhat leathery look. Collagen and elastic fibres in the dermis (the deeper skin layer) become damaged by chronic sun exposure and eventually the skin will become a slightly yellowy colour and start to wrinkle. This occurs over and above the normal changes related to chronological ageing of the skin. You can clearly see the effect of the sun on your own skin by comparing the skin on the outside (sun exposed side) and the inside of your forearm. The inside of the forearm represents chronological (intrinsic) skin ageing and the outside chronological plus photo-ageing. It can be quite sobering to see what the sun has done over time.

I often hear people saying they are going to get a nice 'base-tan' using a sunbed before they go abroad on holiday. They hope that this will help to protect their skin from sunburn whilst they are on a sunny holiday. To an extent, I can understand the logic behind this. Yes, if you have very pale skin and are liable to develop sunburn then having some melanin granules in your skin (a tan) before you go away will make you less likely to get sunburn. However, to achieve this you have had to expose yourself to sunbed UV. Research has shown that although this may result in less sunburn, overall there is a much higher UV exposure and therefore accumulation of more photo-damage in the skin.

If you have a darker skin tone then you are less vulnerable to the damage from UV light and less likely to develop skin cancer, and any tanning is less likely to cause any harm.

So what about if you do still want to get a tan, are sunbeds and fake tan safe?

Sunbeds are made up of lots of fluorescent tubes which emit ultraviolet radiation (UVR). The type and amount of UVR coming out of the tubes is highly variable depending on the type of tube, the age of the tubes and how close the tubes are to your skin.

Professor Elliott, a consultant clinical physicist at the University of Glasgow, has been advising the UK government about the effects of UVR on human health. He reported that research papers show that people who use sunbeds increase their risk of developing melanoma (a cancerous mole) by 59% if they use them within the first 30 years of their life. This is rather worrying, as studies have shown that 82% of sunbed users are under the age of 35. So the very people who are most at risk from the harmful effects of sunbeds, are the people most likely to use them.

The World Health Organisation (WHO) has recommended that people should not use sunbeds under the age of 18 years and should not exceed two sessions per week for a maximum 30 weeks per year. Even this sound like quite a lot considering that most courses of therapeutic artificial light prescribed by doctors (to treat severe psoriasis or eczema) consist of 2-3 times per week for only 8-12 weeks. And the fluorescent tubes used in these phototherapy units are highly regulated and monitored, unlike in some tanning studios.

What everyone does at least agree on, is that younger people are more vulnerable to the effects of sunbeds and solar radiation because their skin is thinner. Consequently, many countries including the UK have now stipulated that it is illegal for those under the age of 18 years to use sunbeds. However, as many tanning salons currently require no proof of age to be shown, stopping those under the age of 18 from using sunbeds is difficult to police. Recently, when a local council in Liverpool conducted a survey of sunbed use, they found that about 40% of sunbed users were in fact under the age of 18.

A new organisation called the Sunbed Association was set up in the UK to ensure that sunbed operators comply with 'best practice'. The problem is however that not all sunbed operators are members of this organisation. Many people believe that until legislation and licencing is linked to compulsory training, monitoring, the provision of safety goggles and available health information then not all operators are prepared to fully comply with best practice.

Even more worryingly, despite safety standards being in place recent studies have shown that the majority of sunbeds give off unsafe levels of UVR. In Scotland for example many tanning salons have now installed new high power sunbeds which emit much higher levels of UVB. Whereas previously it was estimated that 10 minutes on a sunbed was equivalent to 10 minutes of sunshine that you would experience in the Mediterranean summer, many of these new high power sunbeds have been found to produce radiation up to six times more powerful than the upper level recommended as safe (i.e. six times more powerful than the Mediterranean summer sun).

At least in Scotland it is now illegal to have unmanned sunbeds, but this is not the case in England where so called 'slot-machine' sunbeds are still in use. In reality this means that anyone of any age could use them as often as they wish. There is evidence from some studies that burns from too much UVR (which are linked to the development of cancerous moles called melanoma) are more common in people using coin-operated machines than in those who visit manned sunbeds.

Regulation of sunbeds is starting to improve in the UK, and eventually we may have robust systems in place to inspect every piece of tanning equipment every two years, as they currently have in France.

Ultimately, whatever the risks are of sunbeds those using them are usually trying to get tanned. Let's look at the way the skin actually develops a tan since the ability of each of us to tan depends on our skin tone or prototype (described by Fitzpatrick as a number between 1-6). Generally, the fairer our skin the more vulnerable we are to sunburn, the less likely we are to get a tan and the more likely we are to develop a skin cancer.

Fitzpatrick Skin Phototypes

Skin Phototype	Typical Skin Appearance	Ability to Tan	Susceptibility to Sunburn/ Skin Cancer
1	White skin, blond/red hair	Never tans	High
2	Fair skin, blue eyes	Tans eventually	High
3	Darker white skin	Tans moderately easily	Moderate
4	Light brown skin	Tans easily	Low
5	Brown skin	Tans very easily	Very low
6	Dark brown/black skin	Tans very easily	Very low

For those with a fair skin the only safe tan, we are told, is a 'fake one'. So what is a fake or 'sunless tan', how does it develop and is it really safe?

Fake tans are achieved when a substance called dihydroxyacetone (DHA) is applied to the skin. DHA is derived from sugar cane, and it's what gives beer its golden-brown colour. The fake tanning effect of DHA was discovered by accident in the 1950s when it was being used to treat children with glycogen defects. A scientist called Eva Wittgenstein noticed that if some of the DHA was spilt it turned the skin an orange colour. DHA was first approved by the FDA in 1977 for its use in fake tanning lotions. Some modern formulations also contain erythrulose, whose bronzing effects take longer to develop than DHA.

How do these chemicals work? Basically, the DHA and/or erythrulose binds to the amino acids (protein units) in the dead keratinocyte layer at our skin surface. This reaction leads to the production of melanoidins in the skin which, over a period of 4-72 hours, darkens the colour of our skin and makes it appear tanned. Interestingly, these melanoidins are the same chemicals produced in meats as they roast in the oven. Unfortunately, when DHA reacts with the skin an odour is produced which has been likened to the smell of biscuits, barbequed bacon or even curry!

But are these naturally occurring chemicals really safe? At the concentrations used in fake tanning products (DHA 3-5% in over the counter preparations or up to 15% in salon sprays) they are thought to be safe. About 11% of the DHA applied is absorbed into the living cells of the skin but since these cells move towards the surface of the skin, they die naturally and with time are shed, so the effects of the chemicals are thought to be negligible. Some scientists are worried about the potential effects of inhaling micro-droplets of DHA when a fake tan lotion is being sprayed on. At the moment, there is no evidence that this causes any harm to humans, but it might be wise to hold your breath whilst fake tan spray is being applied.

But the most important thing to realise is that the melanoides are not protective. In other words, a fake tan does not protect you from the sun (in fact there is some evidence you might even be a bit more sensitive to sunlight initially) so you will still need to be careful in the sun. Some fake tan lotions also contain sunscreen but that will only last a few hours whereas the fake tan will usually last about 10 days.

So, the effects of sun induced tanning can last a lot longer than the brown colour of our skin and we need to try to limit the amount of intense sun we expose ourselves to if we have fair vulnerable skin. Avoiding sunburn is always thought to be sensible and ensuring we have sufficient vitamin D from the sun alone is a challenge even living in sunny climates. Fake tans appear to be safe, but they can be a challenge to apply evenly and don't protect us from the sun.

Top Tips of Tanning

- Avoid sunbeds if under the age of 18 years.

- If you feel you need to use a sunbed check your provider is a member of the Sunbed Association.

- Always wear eye protection/sunglasses if using a sunbed or out on a sunny day.

- Protect your vulnerable skin from sunburn, especially face, neck and shoulders.

- Avoid the 'leathery ageing effect' of chronic sun exposure by using regular sun protection.

- If you want to look tanned, consider using a fake tan as it's much safer.

CHAPTER 3

Sun Protection, What Works?

What should we do to protect ourselves from the sun? Is sitting in the shade sufficient? Which are the most vulnerable areas of our skin for sun-damage? Are sunscreens safe?

In chapters 1 and 2 we explored the beneficial and harmful effects of ultraviolet radiation (UVR) on our skin during the course of our lives, and what happens during tanning. We know that those effects from the sun can accumulate with time and that we are most vulnerable when we are young. So how can we limit the damage to our skin whilst still reaping the benefits of the sun?

Generally, we need to avoid sunburn as this is thought to be the most destructive form of damage to our skin from strong sunlight. The two main types of UVR from which we need to protect our skin are UVB (290-320nm) and UVA (320-400nm). UVB has a shorter wavelength and penetrates the skin less deeply than

UVA. In general terms, UVB is the burning type of UVR and is present at high levels in the summer months and at its greatest intensity in the middle of the day. This is the type of UVR that is thought to be responsible for most skin cancer and sun damage to the skin.

UVA, on the other hand, is the ageing (wrinkling) sort of UVR that maintains the same intensity throughout the year and throughout the day. It can pass through both clouds and glass so we are pretty much bathed in UVA during daylight hours, whether we are inside or outside. There is increasing evidence however that UVA may also have a role to play in the development of skin cancer. So protection against both UVB and UVA is probably best.

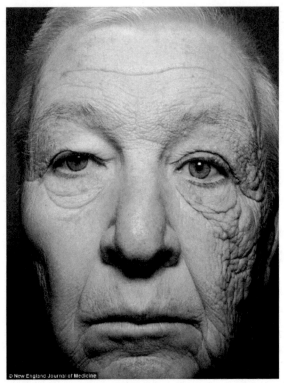

Sun damage on left side of face (window side) truck driver.

This striking photo (reproduced here with permission from *New England Journal of Medicine*) shows the sun-damaged (older looking) skin on the left side of this trucker's face after many years driving a left-hand drive vehicle, compared to the relatively photo-protected (younger looking) right side.

So, what measures can we take to help protect ourselves from the damaging effects of strong sunlight? Many of us will have heard that we should sit in the shade to protect ourselves from the midday sun. But does this mean that we are really protected from the sun's harmful rays? Is it possible that sitting under a tree in the shade means we are 'out of the sun'?

When you stroll through the park on a sunny summer day you can see all the sun-seekers stretched out on the grass in full sunlight, with as much skin exposed as possible (hopefully without offending too many passers-by!), with the aim of getting tanned. Whereas the cautious folk (like me - well, what do you expect from a dermatologist!?) are all sitting in the shade enjoying the outdoors without the 'burn'. But how much are we really protected by sitting in the shade – well, the answer is 'it depends' on what is providing the shade.

Not all shade is equal! It's not surprising to hear that trees with dense foliage are more protective than trees with sparse foliage, as shown in a study conducted in Australia by Gies and colleagues in 2007. But like others, these researchers also found that there are many other variables that affect how much UV protection a tree provides. Larger more mature trees with wide canopies give the most protection against direct sunlight. However, before you rush out and sit under your nearest old oak tree there are other factors found to play a role: height of the tree, changing elevation of the sun with the season and global latitude. Sunlight may also be diffuse or reflected as well as direct. For example, the ground surface under a tree can affect how much light is reflected back up. Manmade concrete surfaces such as pavements and tarmac reflect three times more light than grass.

UVR reflectance from different surfaces.

Surface	% sunlight reflected back
Natural grass	1-4%
Calm (rough) water	3-8% (8-13%)
Concrete	7-12%
Sand	15-18%
Snow	85-88%

So, does the type of tree itself matter? Diffey and colleagues in the UK looked at common UK tree species to see if the type of tree you sat under made a difference. They compared deciduous (all the leaves fall off in the winter) with evergreen (leaves stay on all year round). The sun protection factor (SPF) of the weeping willow (deciduous) was 4 whereas the beech tree (also deciduous) scored 20. Protection was related to the size and density of the leaves. They also measured SPF sitting in the peripheral shade of a Douglas fir (evergreen) which scored 8 and then took the measurement again, but this time next to the trunk and found a SPF or 50! Which is a big difference for just a few feet away.

In other words, there is not much difference between deciduous and evergreen trees, but how deep you sit in its shade does matter. Just watch out when sitting next to tree trunks in case there are any 'deposits' from passing dogs! Just another factor to consider when picking the right spot for that summer picnic (no one said it was going to be easy!) Not surprisingly, if you go into a wooded or forested area the SPF can be up to 100, so ultra-protection from the overlapping canopies, but you might find it a little cold even on a sunny day in temperate climates.

The good news is that these studies also showed that trees were just as good at protecting you from the sun as man-made purpose built shade structures. Local councils can feel reassured in the knowledge that they are helping the environment and local residents by planting trees in communal areas. So the answer is, no, you're not out of the sun when you sit in the shade but it definitely gives you some passive protection from sunburn and sun damage to your skin. Best trees to sit under are mature ones with a wide canopy and sit towards the centre of the shade, nearer to the trunk than the periphery.

Whether it's on the beach or by the pool, many people bring or hire an umbrella/parasol to sit under. But, how protective is that? Sitting under an umbrella with the sun directly overhead can be highly protective from direct sunlight (virtually 90-95%) but only about 60% protective against diffuse sunlight. But at midday

85% of sunlight is in the direct beam form and only 15% is diffuse (scattered) sunlight. So sitting under an umbrella is very helpful – but it's not complete protection from the sun.

What do you do if there are no trees/umbrellas or other shade providing structures around? Then you'll need to get proactive and use clothing such as hats, long sleeves, sunglasses and sunscreen. So how protective are hats? Ones with a brim are definitely the most protective for those vulnerable bits of our face, such as the tops of our ears and the nose, but to give proper protection they need to have a brim of at least 3 inches – so they may not be the best fashion statement, but having portable shade does have its advantages! At least you can get out from under your tree or umbrella! A study conducted in Australia by Gies and colleagues (2006) looked at the protection to the face provided by different types of hat. Bucket, broad-brimmed, cap and Legionnaire style hat. They looked at the protection provided to the forehead, cheek, nose, ears and neck by the different styles of hat in strong overhead sunlight. Legionnaire style hats with the flaps at the sides and back were very successful at protecting the ears and neck. Broad brimmed and bucket hats gave excellent protection to the forehead, nose and ears. The table shows data from Gies paper indicating the Protection Factor (PF) achieved on specific sites on the face/neck by the different types of hats.

Hat Style	Forehead	Cheek	Nose	Ears	Neck
Brimmed	16	2.5	6.8	8.2	2.3
Bucket	15	2.2	6.7	8.1	2.2
Legionnaires	13	1.6	10	4.6	4.3
Caps	8.8	1.1	4.6	1.1	1.3

Baseball type caps are hugely popular worldwide: however, they were the least photoprotective type of hat tested in the study and were particularly poor at protecting the ears. The ears are third commonest site for the most prevalent form of skin cancer, called basal cell carcinoma (40% in front of the ear, 36% on the back of the ear and 24% on the rim of the ear). So if you're wearing a cap remember to put sunscreen on your ears!

For those of us with finer hair or those who are starting to 'thin a little on top' we will certainly benefit from a natty hat, as the UVR tends to beat straight down on the top of our heads and can cause a lot of damage over time. Recent studies (2015) looking at the photo-protection offered by hair (yes, dedicated scientist de Galvez studied this), found that increasing hair density, hair thickness and higher levels of melanin (pigment) were the most protective against UVR. But most of us don't have much control over our hair type/density.

Another part of your photo-protective fashion statement could be clothing with long sleeves to cover the 'sunny side' of your arms. Which is the 'sunny side'? Well, if you look at your arm you can soon see which is the 'sunny side' and which is the 'shady side'. It can be quite telling to look at the inner underside of your arm; this is what your skin looks like for your age without sun changes. Most people with fair skin have freckles, moles and pigmentation on the 'sunny side' of their arm with virtually nothing on the other side. It can be quite interesting and at times sobering to see so starkly what the sun has done to our skin over the years.

Many people believe that they are born with freckles. Well, that's a myth, you are not. Freckles appear over time and are almost always linked to past sun exposure in someone genetically susceptible with fair skin. Freckles are particularly marked after episodes of sunburn, when redness (and at times blisters) settle, the skin heals with distinct areas of freckles that mark the spot for many years to come.

Long sleeves can certainly help to keep that sunny side of our arms protected in the midday sun. But just like hats, not all long sleeves are the same as it depends on the density of the weave and the thickness of the material from which the clothing is made. A study conducted in 2011 by a French group (Ghazi and colleagues), looked at the photo-protection provided by clothing for children under the age of three years. They measured the thickness and UVR protection of different articles of clothing. The sun protection offered by clothing is measured in UV-protection factor (UPF). They found that jeans, tracksuits, sweatshirts, pullovers and tights were highly protective with UPF's of greater than 500.

However, it is unlikely that parents will dress their toddlers in these articles of clothing on a sunny summer's day. In fact parents are more likely to choose short sleeved T-shirts or cotton shirts for their children in sunny weather and these articles gave much lower levels of protection, around UPF 10. Interestingly, the darker colours gave more protection from the sun than lighter colours. A T-shirt of the same thickness material in white gave a UPF score of 12 whereas in black it gave 70. Again, not many parents probably choose black for their three-year-old for summer wear. And what about the heat absorption of dark colours, I hear you cry! Quite right: white reflects heat and dark absorbs heat so we have to consider not causing children to overheat in the sun. So it's all a bit of a conundrum. Special UV protective clothing is available to buy for children and adults and the advanced technology means they now pretty much look like regular clothes.

Most of us will stick to cool clothing (in both senses of the term) and rely more on sunscreen to protect us from the sun. Well, unlike clothing which provides constant sun protection at the same levels for hours on end, sunscreen effects can wear off as time passes, requiring reapplication throughout the day. But how many of us do that?! We will always 'apply' our clothes before we go out but do we always 'apply' our sunscreen? A fair question. Many a time I have forgotten to apply sunscreen or I have underestimated the power of the sun until it's too late.

And if you thought photo-protective clothing was confusing in terms of what to wear, sunscreen is even more challenging! Sun protection factor (SPF) refers to the UVB protection provided by a sunscreen and the star rating (or number in some cases) protection against UVA. SPF is basically telling you how effective a sunscreen is at protecting you against sunburn. So what do the numbers on the sides of the bottles actually mean? A recent survey by the Royal Pharmaceutical Society found that out of the 2000 UK adults they asked, one in four said they did not know what the SPF rating stood for, and only one in three checked for UVA protection when buying sunscreen.

So what does it all mean? If without sunscreen you usually burn after 10 minutes when out in strong sunlight, then after you apply SPF 15 then it will take 15 times longer before you burn, which is 150 minutes. You might logically think therefore that a sunscreen with SPF 30 will give you twice as much protection as SPF 15. Well yes and no! It will take 30 times longer to burn but it filters out 97% of UVB whereas SPF 15 filters out 93%. That's because the relationship between protection and SPF is not a linear one, but a curve. In other words they are both highly protective from sunburn.

How is the SPF number calculated? Well, without getting too technical, 2mg of sun cream is spread over $1cm^2$ of skin (size of a postage stamp) and a certain amount of UVB/UVA is irradiated onto the skin for a fixed amount of time. The more protective of the skin the sunscreen is in this test the higher the number/star rating of the preparation. A study recently conducted by the UK consumer watchdog 'Which?' found most sunscreens offered the level of protection indicated on the side of the bottle, but a couple did not. But in 'real life' do we apply the sunscreen in the way it is tested in the laboratory?

Unfortunately, most of the evidence suggests that we don't. We actually apply between 0.5-1mg/cm^2 and therefore achieve about ½ to 1/3rd of the labelled protection value number/star rating indicated on the label. Therefore the number on the bottle could be misleading. So why don't we change the way that the test is done to reflect more what happens in reality and change the sunscreen labelling accordingly? Well, this has been debated at a global level and the experts all think that this would confuse us even more, so for the moment the current testing and labelling remains.

So what level of SPF/UVA protection do I actually need? Well, you won't be surprised to hear that 'it depends'. Firstly you need to decide how your skin (or indeed your children's skin) reacts to the sun. Ask yourself these questions: If I go out into strong (intense) sunlight without sunscreen how does my exposed skin react? Do I always burn and never tan? (Type I skin – on the Fitzpatrick scale, you will usually have red/auburn/blond hair and blue eyes, freckles); do I usually burn but can get a bit of a tan eventually? (Type II, fair hair, green/blue/hazel eyes); do I occasionally burn but tan relatively easily? (Type III, fair hair, eye colour any); do I rarely burn and always tan very readily? (Type IV, Mediterranean type brown skin tone); do I very rarely burn and tan very easily? (Type V, dark brown skin tone); or do I never burn and always tan very easily? (Type VI, deeply pigmented skin tone).

This tells you your level of in-built protection from the sun, from zero (Type I) to 100% protection (Type VI). If you are of skin type I-III then you need to be more careful in strong sunlight than if you have skin type IV-VI. For those with skin type I-III who are going out on a sunny day, particularly where the sun is very strong (as in the tropics/southern hemisphere), then applying sunscreen to exposed skin areas is advisable. That sunscreen should ideally contain protection against UVB and UVA, these sunscreens are referred to as broad or multi-spectrum.

So what about the actual chemicals used in the sunscreens? And are all broad spectrum sunscreens basically the same? Chemicals that give good multi-spectrum (UVA and UVB) cover include zinc oxide (ZnO), titanium dioxide (TiO_2), avobenzone, oxybenxzone, sulisobenzone, cinnamates and ecamsule.

These chemical names can sound quite alarming especially if you are applying them to the skin of young children, so are they really safe to use? The chemicals are termed 'filters' and they are classified as organic or inorganic. Organic filters are aromatic (ring-shaped) structures that offer protection by absorbing UV light. They absorb harmful high energy UVR and convert it to less harmful lower energy infrared light which is then emitted (sent back out) from the skin. The inorganic filters by contrast reflect the UVR by scattering the light away from the skin.

There have been a number of controversies about the safety of organic and inorganic filters over the past decade. Some early studies suggested that the absorbing organic filters might interfere with hormones in the body, however all the subsequent studies pretty much agree that organic filters are not absorbed into the body in any meaningful amounts and are non-accumulative. Researchers estimate for example that the organic filter oxybenzone would need to be applied daily for more than 300 years to achieve levels in the body that could affect the hormones oestrogen and androgens. Some individuals do develop an allergy to organic filters, but this is true of virtually any chemical applied to the skin.

Inorganic filters include TiO_2 and ZnO which are more photo-stable and less photo-allergic than the organic filters. However recently the safety of inorganic filters has also come into question because newer formulations have been produced using nanoparticle technology. This is the production of incredibly tiny particles (<100nm) of a substance (that's one ten thousandths of a millimetre). The advantage of the nanoparticles of TiO_2 and ZnO is that because they are ultra-small they are more transparent when they are applied to the skin, so they don't leave a white surface residue. Initially there were concerns that these tiny particles might travel into the skin: however, there is no evidence from any studies so far that this happens. There have also been concerns about the workers themselves inhaling these tiny particles during the manufacturing process, but to date there is no evidence that these nanoparticles lead to lung disease.

A study conducted by Ghazi in 2011 looked at the effectiveness of sunscreens especially manufactured for children. They found that only the sunscreens that combined both the organic and inorganic filters gave a SPF of 50+. Inorganic filters TiO_2 and ZnO were found to be equally protective against UVA, but TiO_2 was more protective than ZnO against UVB. You will remember that UVB is at higher levels in the summer months and is responsible for burning and therefore it's the one we really need to protect against. So, the consensus appears to be stick to using reflective inorganic filters for babies and young children, which are not absorbed and yet give very high levels of protection. And frankly if I am buying sunscreen for my kids then I am going to use the same stuff – one bottle for the whole family, simple! Also, look out for offers in the shops of 'buy one get one free' then there will be plenty to go around. You might like to consider buying Altruist Dermatologist Sunscreen online, which is highly effective, rubs in easily, is hypoallergenic, relatively inexpensive and helps support people in Africa who have albinism (reduced skin pigment).

You may have heard of the highly-publicized study a few years ago, that seemed to suggest that those who wore higher factor sunscreens were more likely to get skin cancer later in life? I just want to put the record straight. What the researchers were actually observing was that people with fair skin are the individuals who are more likely to apply high factor sunscreen if they were going out in intense sunlight and for prolonged periods. And hey presto! This is the same combination of factors that cause skin cancer – fair skin, high intense ultraviolet and prolonged exposure. The study even showed that people stayed out much longer than they would have done if they applied low levels or no sunscreen. In other words, because they felt 'extra protected' they stayed out in the sun for longer. It is these risk factors and our behaviours that lead to skin cancer and not high factor sunscreen.

Some people use sunbeds before going on a sunny holiday to try to get a 'base tan' in the hope that this will prevent them from getting sunburn later. This thinking process is understandable: however, overall they are exposing themselves to much more UVR. It is very difficult to know how much UVB and UVA you are being exposed to from a sunbed as there are many variables such as the type of light tubes, the age of the tubes and how close they are to your skin. These people tend to have very strong sun seeking behaviour and are aiming to get tanned, so overall they are increasing their risk for skin cancer and certainly skin ageing (wrinkling).

How should sunscreen be applied? Ideally it should be applied before going out into the sun and to all the exposed skin. Try not to miss any bits and if necessary ask someone to help you apply cream to your back. The timing of reapplication will depend on lots of factors but particularly think of loss of effectiveness if you are sweating a lot or going in and out of water. The definition of water resistant is that the sunscreen should still be effective after 40 minutes in water and very water resistant as still effective after 80 minutes of swimming. So not bad, but not waterproof and it will still need to be reapplied.

All this sounds quite complex and a bit of a mission, but it will be worth it in the end. Bear in mind that most skin cancer is now preventable with the knowledge we have, and that photoprotection will keep our skin looking much younger for longer. Most cosmetic surgeons recommend sunblock as the single most effective anti-ageing product!

Top Sun Protection Tips

• Apply sunscreen containing inorganic filters (Titanium dioxide and Zinc oxide) to any skin that will be exposed, 15-30 minutes before going out into the sun.

• Apply sunscreen generously (about two tablespoons to cover an adult).

• Reapply sunscreen every two hours, take into account SPF, sun intensity, water/sweat.

• Check your sunscreen is not out of date, once opened shelf life is about 18 months.

- Apply sunscreen before applying insect repellent, especially if using organic sunscreen filters.

- Wear a dark coloured thick weave broad-brimmed hat.

- Sit near the trunk of a mature tree with a wide canopy to get the best shade.

- Try to avoid the burning midday sun (between 11am and 2pm ideally).

- Don't forget sunglasses, UVR can damage your eyes leading to cataracts.

CHAPTER 4

Acne, Why Have I got it?

Is the term 'teenage acne' misleading? Does eating too much chocolate give us spots? Can we really cause scarring by squeezing? What's the best treatment for acne?

'Spots' or 'break-outs' are known in medical terms as acne, which is a very common condition. It is estimated that 80% of the population will have acne at some point in their lives. Often acne starts in the teenage years, hence the reference to 'teenage spots'. However, many people find that term misleading, as it suggests after the teenage years the acne should resolve. The current reality is that acne that starts in the teens can continue into the 20s, 30s and even the 40s. For example, at age 45 years 5% of the population still suffers from acne. So, what actually causes spots?

There is no doubt that the tendency to have acne is related in part to genetics. Acne tendencies can run in the family, with a father and/or mother passing down the 'acne' genes to their children. Certain ethnic groups, such as those living in the Mediterranean, often suffer from a more severe cystic form of the condition, called nodulocystic acne, which is more likely to result in permanent scarring. Your natural skin tone can also affect how the acne looks and behaves. For example, those with naturally darker skin tones are more likely to have pigmentation marks on their skin after the acne settles (so-called post-inflammatory hyperpigmentation) which can stay for many months. There is also a slight variation between the sexes. In adolescence boys are more commonly affected than girls but in adulthood it is more common in women than in men.

So how does acne start? As a general rule the majority of acne starts when our sex organs start to produce more androgen hormones around the time of puberty. Androgens trigger an increase in sebum production (the natural grease of the skin) within sebaceous (grease) glands. There is an inflammatory response where lots of active chemicals called cytokines are released around the sebaceous glands and this combination of events leads to plugging of the hole where the gland and the hair come out onto the skin (the sebaceous/follicular opening or pore). We see this plugging as comedones, which are very small bumps on the skin that can feel like rough grains of sand. They are commonly called 'black heads' (open comedones) or 'white heads' (closed comedones), which are blocked or partially blocked sebaceous gland openings. The black colour is not dirt as some people think, it's actually melanin pigment within the opening that in contact with the air has been oxidised, causing the dark colour.

The increase in cytokines and increased sebum production inside the sebaceous glands causes an increase in the numbers of *Propionibacterium acnes* (*P. acnes*) bacteria which in turn lead to an increase in skin inflammation, basically a 'vicious cycle'. What we see on our skin as a result of all this is enlarged pores, redness (inflammation), swelling (bumps), pustules (collections of inflammatory cells and sebum) and eventually cysts (completely blocked sebaceous glands that don't come to a 'head'). Not everyone will have all the different types of acne lesions at the same time, but as a general rule acne starts with comedones and then progresses to inflammatory and pustular spots and then finally to nodulo-cystic lesions. The latter are deep in the skin and can remain for months or years, and it is these lesions that are most likely to lead to permanent acne scarring.

So what about the other factors that might play a role in stimulating or worsening our acne? It has been suggested in the past that body mass index, glucose levels, emotional stress, make-up, pollution, insufficient skin cleaning and diet may also play a role in acne in addition to our background genetics and hormone levels.

Foods commonly suspected of playing a role in acne include fatty foods, dairy products, milk and chocolate. In my experience, many acne sufferers will say that they notice that if they eat chocolate or sugary/fatty foods that their acne spots become worse. As a general principle, I recommend that if anything seems to exacerbate any skin condition, then if possible the offending trigger should be avoided as much as possible. But is there actually a proven link between food and acne?

There have been several publications showing that populations who eat a non-Westernised diet don't suffer from acne. A Westernised diet is thought to be generally lacking in omega-3 and high in refined carbohydrates. A recent study in Australian men looked at the link between the glycemic index (GI) of the foods they ate and their acne. Carbohydrate rich foods increase our blood sugar levels either quickly (high glycemic index, >70) or slowly (low glycemic index, <55). High GI foods include white bread, white rice, most breakfast cereals and potatoes and low GI foods include vegetables, beans/pulses and nuts/whole grains. High GI foods not only raise blood sugar levels quickly, they also elevate serum insulin levels (which may stimulate sebum production), and there is evidence insulin also increase androgen levels.

In this Australian study 43 males with acne aged between 15-25 years were recruited for a three-month period. Half the group were told to follow a strict low GI diet and the other group were told to have carbohydrate-dense food (with no mention of GI factors). Acne lesion counts and severity were assessed for the two groups (in addition to their insulin sensitivity). The low GI group had less acne and less severe acne than the other group at the end of the three months. Interestingly, they had also lost some weight and their sensitivity to insulin had improved. So this study does suggest a link between diet and acne, but it's not conclusive (as weight and insulin sensitivity also changed). In addition, only small numbers of male patients participated, but nonetheless the results are interesting. However, if eating foods with a high GI index and reduced insulin sensitivity leads to acne, why don't most overweight individuals suffer from spots? There is still more research needed for us to fully understand the GI index of food and its possible links to acne.

What about the observation that many people make between eating chocolate and exacerbation of their acne? A recent study recruited 14 males between the ages of 18-35 years with mild acne and they were asked to swallow capsules (all in one dose) containing either unsweetened 100% cocoa, hydrolysed gelatin powder (amino acids) or a combination of both. Acne lesions were assessed before the start and during the one week period following the dose taken, using photographs. There was an increase in the number of acne lesions (comedones and inflammatory pustules) seen at day 4 and day 7 which correlated with the amount of unsweetened chocolate capsules consumed. So this slightly goes against the idea that it must be the sugar in the chocolate that is the trigger for acne. Indeed, if we believe that low GI is associated with less acne then chocolate should be OK as it's actually a relatively low GI food. Dark chocolate (with a cocoa content >70%) has a GI index of 23 and milk chocolate has a GI of 34-49, so higher than dark chocolate but still relatively low.

So maybe it's something else that is contained within cocoa that is the potential trigger?

A Korean study conducted by Kwon and colleagues in 2012 looked at low glycaemic index diet and sebaceous gland size, and found they tended to shrink and consequently subjects had less acne.

What about dairy products and milk? The possible link between dairy and acne has been debated for years but unfortunately no real definitive answer has been forthcoming. This may be because most of the studies were based on questionnaires which asked people to recall how much and what type of dairy products (particularly cow's milk) they consumed in the past and what their skin was like at the time in terms of acne lesions. This type of recall can be pretty unreliable, but most studies seemed to suggest that higher milk consumption is associated with more acne. But what is it about the milk that can affect acne? A recent publication reports the development of acne for the first time in 5 healthy males who took whey protein to help them with bodybuilding. Whey protein is made up of amino acids and is derived from milk where the casein has been separated from the whey. So this may add to the suggestion that milk can exacerbate/cause acne.

Researchers have recently pointed to milk being a possible cause of some individual's exacerbation of acne. Adebamowo and colleagues studied over 6000 girls and over 4000 boys and followed them for 3 years – their studies show there is a weak link between drinking milk and having acne. Interestingly skimmed milk seemed to be just as bad as full fat milk in terms of acne stimulating and acne aggravating, so the fat content of the milk didn't seem to the be key factor.

Another recent observational study of 115 males and 133 females between the ages of 18-25 years in the USA asked participants to complete food diaries and self-report on their acne severity. Bearing in mind recall of diet and self-assessed skin lesions, there did seem to be more severe acne reported with greater dietary GI, dietary sugar, milk servings, saturated fat, trans-fatty acids and fewer portions of fish per day. Interestingly 58% of those taking part in the study felt that diet did influence their acne.

The so-called Palaeolithic diet is a very fashionable and modern diet thought to promote healthy eating and reduce our chance of developing diabetes. This diet is based on eating low glycaemic index foods, no milk and no dairy. A couple of randomised controls trials showed that those on the PD had less acne than those on a normal diet. So again some suggestion that dairy might be acne-promoting. So it may be worth advising young teenagers with mild acne to try reducing the amount of milk they consume and stick to low glycaemic index foods to help settle their acne more quickly or indeed to try to prevent it becoming more severe.

So where does this leave us in our understanding about diet and acne? There is no doubt that more research is needed in this area, but based on what we know at present it would seem sensible to try to follow a low GI diet and don't drink large quantities of milk if you suffer from acne. There is no doubt that a diet that limits high sugar and saturated fat intake can help us to remain at a healthy weight and lower our risk of diabetes and heart disease so it's probably a sensible approach to take whether you suffer from acne or not.

Some experts have also pointed to the potential links between vitamins A/D and acne. Vitamin A derivatives (retinoic acid, tretinoin, isotretinoin) as cream and as tablet formulations have been used for many years to treat acne. So what is the link between vitamin A/D and acne? *P. acnes* the bacteria that proliferate around the sebaceous glands in acne are partly responsible for increasing the inflammation in acne skin. *P. acnes* achieve this by triggering some T-lymphocytes in the skin (T-helper 17 cells) – which are part of our white cell population and this then triggers a cascade of inflammation. Vitamin A and D have been shown to inhibit this trigger of T-helper cells by *P. acnes*, thus reducing inflammation. A recently published study found that when 94 patients with acne had their serum levels of vitamins checked they were found to have significantly lower levels of vitamin A, E and zinc when compared to healthy age-matched controls.

Hormones may also play a role in acne, and unlike diet, may be more difficult to control. Some women suffer from polycystic ovarian syndrome (PCOS) which is an endocrine condition where there is a slight imbalance in some hormone levels (usually increased levels of androgens, testosterone and dehydroepiandrosterone) plus multiple cysts in their ovaries (seen on ultrasound). These women usually have irregular menstrual cycles and frequently have ongoing and quite severe acne (often over the jawline). They may also suffer from hirsuitism (an increase in facial hair), infertility, weight-gain and type 2 diabetes). One treatment that has been shown to help acne in PCOS is a medicine that is also used to treat diabetes, called metformin, which helps the body to regulate blood sugar levels. Interestingly in PCOS some studies have found that if the patients ate a low carbohydrate diet their hormone imbalance also improved. So looking at factors that affect acne in PCOS there does seem to be some sort of link between hormones, blood sugar levels and acne.

Acne has some physical effects on those who are suffering from it, such as painful lesions, tight feeling in the skin, burning discomfort and scarring marks. However, it is the psychological effects that can often be the most debilitating, such as lack of self-esteem, embarrassment, depression (even suicidal thoughts), anxiety and lack of self-confidence and consequently, to reduce the visible impact of acne, many sufferers will try to cover the spots with make-up such as concealers.

But does this 'cover-up' make the acne worse? As a general rule any oil-based occlusive preparations could result in more blocking of the skin pores, which could make the acne worse. Most acne sufferers tend to have an oily skin type and therefore avoid oily preparations on their skin. The skin's normal moisture layer is made up of lipid (oil) and water so although acne patients may have plenty of oil, they may have low levels of water and therefore their skin can feel dry: so-called 'combination skin'. So generally, acne sufferers benefit from more watery gel-type moisturising preparations (rather than the oily ones), which wouldn't block their pores.

Make-up is often sold with labelling suggesting it can be used in 'acne-prone' skin or that it is non-comenogenic (in other words shouldn't induce comedones) so these are a good choice for those of us with an oily skin who have a tendency to develop acne. Powder type foundation is usually a better choice than a creamy one, and make-up should be removed at night using a non-oily make-up remover and warm water. If these simple guidelines are followed then there is no suggestion that using make-up to cover up the acne spots will make the situation worse, and indeed covering up the spots can help to reduce the psychological impact of the condition.

As well as covering up their acne some sufferers will understandably try to 'disrupt' their spots. They will try to unblock the pores and disperse the collections of pus at the surface. This can be achieved at home by using facial scrubs and/or squeezing the spots. If we gently disrupt the top of an acne spot, just removing the pus by wiping, this seems to be reasonably helpful, but as soon as pressure is added in the form of squeezing spots, then damage can occur. The pressure around the sides of the spot can cause the sebaceous gland to partially rupture its sebum contents not only out onto the skin surface but also into the deeper levels of the skin (dermis) which results in an inflammatory response and ultimately scarring. This can leave small permanent indentations sometimes called 'ice-pick' scarring (as it looks as if small deep cuts have been made) on the affected skin. Most skin experts will agree that treating acne in its active form is more straightforward than treating acne scars.

With this in mind some acne sufferers will instead undertake more formal physical treatments such as chemical peels or facials often performed by a practitioner. But is there any evidence that these kinds of physical treatments can help? A recent study looked at the efficacy of applying 40% glycolic acid (GA, chemical peel) to one half of the face versus placebo on the other half in 26 patients with moderate acne. The procedure was performed five times at fortnightly intervals. Neither the patients nor the doctors conducting the study knew which side was treated with which application (double-blinded) until the results were analysed. There were statistically less of the comedonal acne lesions on the GA treated side of the face compared to the placebo half at 10 weeks. But there was no difference in inflammatory acne lesions or lowering of sebum levels comparing the two groups. So physical treatments do help to unblock and clear comedones but don't really help to get rid of the inflammatory pustules.

Microdermabrasion (particle resurfacing) has also increased in popularity over the last 10 years as a minimally invasive cosmetic procedure including treatment for acne/acne scarring. It is estimated in the

USA that about 900,000 cases were performed in 2007. This technique involves using abrasive substances that are blown onto the skin and then vacuumed off again. But is there any evidence it helps in acne? Aluminium oxide or sodium chloride (salt) crystals are often used as the abrasive substance. Examining treated skin histologically by looking down the microscope shows little actual abrasion of the skin and minimal surface change. However there is some evidence that this technique can affect the deeper tissue (the dermis) and does seem to help in skin damaged by photo-ageing.

Studies looking at the effects of microdermabrasion in the treatment of active acne were initially encouraging, however on closer inspection some of these studies were poorly designed, with no control groups. Recent more rigorous split-face studies have shown no benefit from microdermabrasion, in fact many of those treated developed worsening acne and did better when switched to a medical treatment such as topical retinoid or oral antibiotic.

So acne is incredibly common and can last for many years and may lead to psychological and physical scarring effects. We may derive some benefit from eating a low GI diet and use products which are non-comeogenic, however eventually we may need some more 'medicalised' treatment. Most acne sufferers will start with some sort of topical (applied to the skin) treatment, and there is good evidence that benzoyl peroxide (can bleach clothing) and topical retinoic acid are helpful at treating mild/moderate acne. These topical preparations can cause some peeling and redness of the skin so this usually limits the percentage/frequency of application that can be tolerated. Some peeling can be helpful as this helps to unblock the pores. Topical antibiotics are often formulated into a product in addition to benzoyl peroxide to provide additional anti-inflammatory effects as well as skin peeling effects, dual action.

Other treatments can include hormonal preparations in women that help to 'even out' hormonal imbalances. For many years the oral contraceptive pill Dianette (cyproterone acetate and ethinylestradiol) has been used for woman with acne for its anti-androgen effects. It can be highly effective at keeping a lid on acne for many years but is usually not recommended for woman over the age of 35 years. Oral antibiotics particularly from the tetracycline group have been used to treat inflammatory acne (in those over the age of 13) for many years. Usually oral antibiotics need to be taken for between three and nine months for a meaningful and lasting effect on the acne.

Finally, if acne doesn't settle with all these other measures then some patients need oral vitamin A in the form of isotretinoin. This is a potent and effective treatment for recalcitrant acne but has more side effects than topical treatment, hormonal therapy and oral antibiotics and therefore is generally reserved for treating severe acne, nodulocystic disease or patients who have failed to respond adequately to other treatments. Isotretinoin works by shutting down the sebaceous glands in the skin by about 90% and consequently dries out the grease. The drying effect is most marked on the lips, which during the treatment can become quite dry, cracked and painful.

Most courses of isotretinoin need to be taken for about six months depending on the daily dose taken. Most dermatologists recommend a dose close to 1mg/kg of the patient's body weight per day after an initial low dose introductory phase over about six weeks. However continual low dose regimes are also recognised as being effective but the courses tend to last a lot longer (one to two years). In order to try to prevent relapse of the acne once the course has finished, a total target dose of 120-150mg of isotretinoin/kg of the patient's weight in total is recommended.

Overall efficacy rates for isotretinoin are in the order of 90% of patients having a complete remission from their acne with some of the remaining 10% having a partial remission. However, relapse rates are quoted as being anywhere between 30-50%. Examining the medical literature in more detail reveals patients are more likely to relapse if they have severe nodulocystic disease, PCOS, younger age or took an insufficient total amount of isotretinoin in the previous treatment course. In these circumstances, some patients may require a second or even third course of oral isotretinon.

Taking isotretinoin for acne, although highly effective, does cause concern for some patients and indeed doctors because of its long list of potentially serious side effects. It's teratogenic (it would damage a baby in the womb) so women should avoid pregnancy whilst they are taking the medication and also for a 'wash-out' period of one to two months afterwards; it can be photo-sensitizing (makes you more sensitive to the sun); causes myalgia (muscle aches) particularly after exercise and in some patients, it can affect their mood or even cause depression. So, it is a medicine that needs to be taken under close supervision from a practitioner who understands the potential adverse events as well as the potential benefits. Overall though it is highly effective and can literally transform lives.

Top Tips for Managing Acne

- Get acne treatment early to prevent scarring and psychological distress.

- Over the counter benzoyl peroxide is effective at treating mild acne.

- If over the counter treatments aren't helping speak to your GP/dermatologist.

- If you suffer from acne it might be worth trying a low GI diet.

- Avoid oily-based creams on the face if you are prone to acne, as they can block pores.

- Avoid squeezing spots, only use gentle surface disruption, if really necessary.

Skin care regime recommended for those prone to or suffering from acne:

- Wash/clean your face twice a day using a cleanser/soap recommended for acne prone skin.

- Apply a light moisturizer with SPF30 in the morning after skin cleansing.

- At night apply medicated acne preparations to the acne-affected skin areas.

- Use this skin care regime regularly to get the benefit.

CHAPTER 5

Anti-Ageing Treatments, Do they Work?

Why do we develop dark circles under our eyes? Why does the skin start to wrinkle with age? Do anti-wrinkle creams actually work? Are chemical peels safe? Are lasers some kind of 'miracle treatment'?

Have you noticed when you are tired that dark circles can appear under your eyes? It's a strange phenomenon that can literally seem to appear overnight. This dark colour is usually temporary, only lasting a few days, but as we get older the dark colour can persist for months or even years. A study published in 2008 asked trained graders to look at 173 facial photographs of Caucasian women and decide if they were young (less than 35 years), middle age (35-50 years) or senior (> 50 years). Interestingly it was the eye area and skin colour uniformity or lack of it that were the main attributes of perceived older age. So could it be when we are tired we really do look older?

Periorbital hyperpigmentation (POH, dark circles under the eyes) occurs in people of all skin types, but those with darker skin tones are more susceptible. Sometimes the condition can appear in multiple family members through the generations. There is evidence from the medical literature that the more permanent type of pigmentation may be a final common pathway of dermatitis (eczema or inflammation in the skin), allergy (to pollens/dusts or skin/eye products), internal illnesses (such as diabetes, liver problems, thyroid disorders) sleep disturbance (usually chronic) or nutritional deficiencies.

My own personal experience of this happened a few years ago when I had a scooter accident and was 'laid-up' for six weeks and as a result I got lots of rest. Interestingly the dark circles under my eyes (that I have most of the time) vanished! Everyone who came to visit me kept commenting on how well I looked. I have also noticed that when colleagues retire from working in the NHS and come back to visit us a few months later, they too have lost the dark circles under their eyes. They look healthier and younger. I'm not exactly saying that the NHS is 'taking it out of us', but what it does show is that lack of sleep does play a role in the appearance of our periorbital skin.

200 patients attending a dermatology clinic in India were assessed in a study looking at the cause and POH. The condition was most prominent in the age group 16-25 years (47%) and in females (81%). In this cohort POH was more common in younger people than older

people. The underlying cause in the majority was considered to be constitutional POH, due to lack of sleep (40%), frequent associated eye rubbing (32%) and 36% irritant eye cosmetics. There was also a high correlation of POH with stress (71%) and family history of the condition (63%).

What is happening when we don't sleep enough that leads to the skin colour change around our eyes? This question is partially answered by another study that looked at 60 healthy Caucasian women who were divided into those who were poor quality sleepers (using a scoring system called the Pittsburg sleep quality index), who slept less than five hours or good quality sleepers who slept for seven to nine hours. Their skin was assessed using a validated tool SCINEXA(TM) that measures extrinsic (external factors) and intrinsic (biological) ageing including the assessment of dark circles under the eyes. They found that good sleepers had lower skin ageing scores and poor sleepers had significantly higher levels of transepidermal water loss (TEWL).

This increased TEWL means their skin was more likely to lose fluid from it due to diminished barrier function in the poor sleepers. When our skin dries out it loses volume (so becomes thinner), sinks slightly (sunken appearance) and becomes more translucent so that the underlying tissue is more visible. Sitting just underneath the skin below our eyes is a muscle called the orbicularis oculi and it is this muscle that becomes more visible through the translucent skin, leading to the appearance of a dark colour under the eyes.

As we age this temporary process of the skin becoming drier and thinner due to lack of sleep can be accentuated by other factors such as chronic dermatitis, diabetes, familial tendency and sun exposure. These superimposed factors lead to the periorbital pigmentation becoming permanent. At this stage a good night's sleep won't reduce the appearance of the dark circles.

Skin biopsy samples taken to compare the dark skin area with normal adjacent skin in a recent study showed the permanent dark colour was caused by increased melanin (brown pigment) in the dermis (the second layer of the skin) and dilated blood vessels. The darker the circles the more melanin there was and the more prominent the dilated blood vessels. So at this stage something structural had changed in the affected skin which led to permanent pigmentation.

Therefore, it's true that a good night's sleep is helpful at keeping away those dark circles and keeping our periorbital skin looking younger. But we all lead busy lives and a good night's sleep might not be possible, so what can we do to help to combat the temporary thinning process? One study enrolled 57 adult Japanese volunteers with dark circles under their eyes and asked them to apply a gel to the affected skin twice a day for eight weeks. The gel contained 2% phytonadione (vitamin K), 0.1% retinol (vitamin A) plus 0.1% vitamin C and E. Digital photographs were taken before and after the treatment and a visual analogue scale used to assess the outcome. 50% of the women had a reduced appearance of POH according to the study results. However, we don't know whether the hydrating effect of the gel base was the main factor or whether the vitamins played any role. It would have been better if they had treated one side with the gel base and the other side with the gel base plus vitamin cocktail. This poor study design means the results are difficult to accurately interpret.

A more recent study conducted in 2012 to assess the effects of topical applications on POH in 124 women ensured their study design was robust. They had a placebo group (without the active ingredient), randomisation of placebo, 1 or 3 galvanic zinc-copper complex in a gel and activating moisturizer and double-blinding (neither the study subjects or the assessors knew which preparation was being used until after all the assessments were complete). Effects were determined by clinical grading, specialised clinical imaging and self-assessments at baseline, 15-30 minutes after the application and at one, two, four and eight weeks. There was a significant improvement in the zinc-copper application groups compared to placebo, suggesting the active ingredients used in this study did add something to the moisturizer to diminish the appearance of the dark circles.

Although these studies showed that creams can help in some cases, many modern treatments involve a much more interventional approach. A glance at the medical literature reporting treatments for dark circles shows outcomes for the use of injections, fat-transfer, chemical peels and laser treatment. So clearly people do seem to be bothered by the appearance of POH and treating them can be a challenge, with multiple modalities used.

The skin around the eyes is also vulnerable to wrinkling which can appear with increasing age. Over exposure of the skin to the effects of the sun, screwing-up our eyes from laughter/squinting and smoking can lead to increased skin wrinkling. A study published in 2015 examined Dutch and English adults (male and female, smokers and non-smokers) and looked at multiple factors that could affect the degree of facial ageing they displayed. It is no surprise that sunbed use/being outside most of the summer/having fair skin all contributed to a higher degree of skin ageing. But the study also found evidence to support previous observations that smoking caused a significant increased degree of facial skin ageing. Smoking was an independent risk factor for skin wrinkling.

Tobacco smoke extract impairs our ability to make normal collagen (the main structural protein in our skin's connective tissue) and it increases the production of tropoelastin and matrix metalloproteinases (which breakdown matrix proteins). Smoking also causes the production of abnormal elastosis material which takes the form of degenerative elastic and collagen fibres. All these effects cause accelerated wrinkling and therefore ageing of the skin. Smokers' skin has also been described as 'citrine' which comes from the French word, citron, meaning lemon. This yellow appearance of the skin which is usually also quite coarse in texture is also seen in fair people with sun-damaged skin.

How can we try to reverse this skin ageing process? Stopping smoking and using high factor sunscreen is a very good starting point to reduce further accelerated skin ageing. The treatment of skin wrinkles is big business in the developed world, particularly in countries where trying to halt or reverse the ageing process is part of the culture. Brazil is emerging as one of countries in Latin America with the highest number of consumers per head of population in the use of anti-ageing products. USA and China remain the countries with the highest demand.

The most commonly used anti-ageing preparation worldwide is still retinoic acid cream and the most studied form is tretinoin. Studies into the effects of topical tretinoin (in 0.025%-0.1% concentrations) have been carried out over the past 40 years, and these have shown significant benefits to both photo-aged and chronologically aged skin. Traditionally these topical retinoids have been used for six to 12 months to get the full benefit. Retinoic acid can be quite irritant to the skin (causing redness and inflammation), particularly in the first few weeks and this tends to limit the concentration used in these preparations. In many countries, topical tretinoin can only be obtained on a prescription usually prescribed by a private practitioner. So, the cosmetics industry has been trying to formulate 'cosmetic' preparations that can be bought over the counter to try to make anti-ageing creams more widely available.

There has been an impression amongst doctors and cosmetic practitioners that these cosmetic preparations are less irritant than prescription treatments and also less effective. Recent studies conducted by cosmetic companies have tried to dispel this myth by conducting head-to-head studies comparing cosmetic and prescription products.

One study conducted in Ohio, USA and funded by consultants working for Procter and Gamble Beauty (who make Olay products, a potential conflict of interest) compared over the counter cosmetic Olay anti-wrinkle products vs prescription 0.02% tretinoin. The trial was set-up with a randomised controlled comparative design. Women with moderate or moderately severe wrinkles around their eyes were randomised to use the cosmetic products or the tretinoin for eight to 24 weeks. The 99 'cosmetic subjects' were asked to use three products (a sunscreen (SPF 30) lotion, an antioxidant moisturiser cream and an anti-wrinkle cream containing 0.3% retinyl propionate) all also containing niacinamide and peptides. They were told to apply the anti-wrinkle cream morning and evening plus the sunscreen product in the morning and the rich emollient cream in the evening. The 'prescription group' (97 women) were asked to use 0.02% tretinoin cream alternate days for the first two weeks plus moisturising SPF 30 sunscreen daily and then after that initial two-week period both creams daily. Fine lines and wrinkles were assessed by expert graders who were 'blinded' to the treatments used. Overall there was a significant improvement in the fine lines and wrinkles in both groups, with no real discernible differences between the cosmetic and the prescription products.

Another study compared over the counter cosmetic formulations containing 0.25%, 0.5% and 0.1% retinol with three commonly prescribed concentrations (0.025%, 0.05% and 0.1%) of tretinoin. This study was conducted by scientists working for SkinMedica (part of the Allergan Company, a potential conflict of interest). They used a randomised, double-blind (neither study subjects nor assessors knew which treatment was being used) and split-face design (comparing retinol on one half of the face and tretinoin on the other half) for the study. 65 women with moderate to severe facial photo-ageing were randomised to three groups. Group 1 (retinol 0.25% vs tretinoin 0.025%), group 2 (retinol 0.5% vs tretinoin 0.05%) and group 3 (retinol 1.0% vs tretinoin 0.1%). The creams were applied for 12 weeks and then the skin assessed (compared to baseline) for fine and coarse lines/wrinkles, skin tone brightness, mottled pigmentation and skin roughness. There was statistically significant improvement in all three groups and no difference in the effects of retinol compared to tretinoin.

So overall there does appear to be evidence that anti-wrinkle creams do help to reduce the appearance of wrinkles on the face, if applied consistently for weeks/months. However, many people are not prepared to wait for months to see the effects or may have more severe photo-ageing changes and these individuals may opt for more interventional treatments using lasers.

Lasers for many people seem like some kind of miracle appliance that is more sophisticated and more effective than conventional conservative medical treatments, but is this really the case?

In most NHS dermatology departments in the UK there are no laser treatments available. The reason for this is that NHS dermatologists are fully qualified medical doctors who are experts in treating skin disease (skin cancer, acute rashes, psoriasis, eczema, acne etc.) rather than carrying out any cosmetic work. One of the exceptions to this in the UK is that some dermatology departments have a 'vascular laser' to treat facial vascular (blood vessel) birthmarks. But essentially skin laser and cosmetic treatments in the UK are mainly in the domain of the private dermatologist or the cosmetic practitioner.

So what cosmetic preparations and treatments do people use to try to combat the damage caused by too much sun or indeed the natural ageing process of their skin? Over the past few decades interest in anti-ageing treatments has grown. The cosmetics industry is a multi-million-pound business in many in resource-rich countries. Women and men in their 40s-70s are the main age group that seek to try to turn back the clock by reversing the signs of ageing of their skin. As we get older, and if we have had more sun in the past than our skin could take, then we may have wrinkles, pigment spots and our skin can start to sag a little. To combat these skin changes there are numerous over the counter creams available, beauty treatments such as microdermabrasion and so-called 'lunchtime treatments' with intense-pulsed light, injections of botox and fillers. And finally some people resort to chemical peels, lasers or cosmetic surgery. Let's explore some of these treatments in more detail. How do they work and are they really safe?

There is no doubt that one of the most effective treatments for facial wrinkles is laser therapy. The term 'laser' is actually an acronym for 'light amplification by stimulated emission of radiation'. These devices were first made about 50 years ago, and now have multiple uses in all sorts of industries. Laser lights are useful because they can emit light 'coherently'. This coherence is both spatial and temporal. What this means is that the light beam can be focussed into a very small spot and can be of a very narrow wavelength. Lasers emit a single colour of light that can, if desired, be pulsed 'on and off'. These properties mean that each laser is designed to emit a different type of light and for skin treatments, target a different cell type or component of our skin. When the laser light hits the target in the skin (the chromophore) energy is released in the form of heat which can lyse (break/damage) the target cells.

Vascular lasers such as the 'pulsed dye laser' for example are used to treat facial vascular birth marks and dilated blood vessels, target the oxygenated red blood cells inside large blood vessels, causing them to lyse. Hair removal lasers target the black pigment in the hair (melanin) leading to thermal heating and lysis of the hair follicle cells. We also have melanin pigment in our skin, so this type of laser treatment works best if the skin is very fair and the hair is very dark (which is not always the case), otherwise the laser can inadvertently damage the skin pigment.

In the treatment of skin wrinkling, carbon dioxide lasers have traditionally been used and these target water which leads to removal (vaporization) of the top layers of the skin. This vaporization is termed 'resurfacing' and can be done to a desired depth. Obviously if you have had the top layer of your skin vaporized then it's going to looks very swollen, red and feel 'raw' for quite a few days afterwards. This type of laser treatment is pretty 'full-on' and patients need to be selected very carefully and need to fully understand the 'downtime' necessary afterwards, plus the potential risks and well as the potential benefits. Laser resurfacing can be extremely effective leading to fewer 'sun spots' and wrinkles afterwards. Most laser specialists recommend high factor sunscreen on the face afterwards for many months.

The relatively long recovery period resulting from laser resurfacing treatments has put off some of those thinking about having anti-ageing treatments for their skin and consequently the development of less invasive approaches to the treatment of skin ageing has expanded. So-called 'lunch- break treatments' have boomed in the past five years, such as soft tissue augmentation, 'fillers'. These have become popular as they can be easily injected into the skin to try to correct loss of volume, wrinkles and sagging hollows.

Hyaluronic acid, which is a naturally occurring substance, is a popular choice of 'filler'. It attracts and holds water resulting in 'filling' and 'lifting' of the skin. Initially bovine-derived (from cows) products were used, so allergy testing on the forearm was necessary prior to facial injection. Because 3% of people developed an allergy to the bovine material, human collagen in the form of a cell line of human fibroblasts started to replace the bovine fillers. More recently rooster-comb avian (chicken) derived fillers and even streptococci bacteria derived ones have become popular. The skill of the practitioner injecting the filler is crucial to the outcome, and if too much is injected an 'inflated cushion' appearance, 'pillow face' can result, however if done carefully by a highly skilled practitioner the results look natural and can literally 'push back' the years. There can be a few days afterwards of redness at the site of the injections, pain and bruising can also occur. Fillers usually last one to two years, meaning that repeat injections are needed to maintain the effects. Many celebrities these days have fillers injected to keep themselves looking young rather than opting for more invasive laser treatments.

Another lunch-time treatment that seems to be very popular is having Botulinum toxin injections. These are injected to try to reduce the appearance of facial wrinkles particularly on the forehead, around the eyes and mouth. Botox is a neurotoxin derived from bacteria, *Clostridium botulinum*, which inhibits the release of acetylcholine (a neurotransmitter chemical) causing temporary paralysis of the affected muscles. Because the muscles are paralysed, facial expressions become blunted and the skin becomes smooth overlying them. Botox paralysis lasts about six months so needs to be repeated to keep the desired effect. Some people feel that those who have had Botox injections look slightly unnatural, as they are unable to show facial expressions in the normal way. It may be difficult for them to look surprised, happy, angry etc.

Nonetheless, for all their potential drawbacks both fillers and Botox injections are very popular and can reduce the appearance of wrinkles. If however the skin is sun-damaged with textural changes and pigmentation, then usually a treatment that alters the skin surface is needed. This is where chemical peels are sometimes used. These chemicals literally damage the top layer of the skin (in a controlled manner), causing it to blister and then peel off (over about 1-2 weeks). Popular chemicals used include alpha and beta-hydroxy acids, trichloroacetic acid and phenol. The type and concentration of chemical used determines the depth of the damage (superficial, medium or deep) and therefore the resulting peel.

The actual chemical peel procedure starts when acetone or alcohol (defatting solvent) is wiped over the skin to be treated, then the peeling solution is applied for the desired time period and then stopped with neutralizing solution. Whatever the depth of the peel the skin is usually quite red afterwards. Immediately post-peel the face can be quite swollen and it may feel uncomfortable. Less commonly cold sores (herpes simplex virus) can be activated, pigmentation and scarring can occur and acne may be triggered. The recovery period can be weeks for a deep peel. So it's a process not to be undertaken lightly and needs to be carried out by someone who knows what they are doing, and usually after a small 'patch test' (testing a small area of skin first with the peeling agent to see the effect, before treating the entire face). There is no doubt though when the skin rejuvenates itself after the peel the sun-damage changes are usually markedly reduced making the skin appear younger.

If all that sounds a bit too much then how about Intense Pulsed Light (IPL)? This has become very popular in beauty salons, but many medical practitioners are sceptical about whether or not it really works. So what is the evidence that IPL improves wrinkles/signs of ageing/sun-damage in the skin? There is a growing body of evidence to support the observation that IPL reduces pigment spots on the skin such as sun spots (solar lentigos) and freckles. There is also recent evidence to suggest that IPL can reduce the appearance of melasma (confluent patches of pigmentation on the face caused by super-sensitivity to sunlight). However, facial rejuvenation aimed at reducing the appearance of wrinkles appears to be less beneficial with IPL than more invasive treatments such as laser and chemical peels. Many people having IPL treatment however are happy with the slow gentle approach to clawing back the effects of sunshine and ageing rather than suffer any down-time after more potent therapies.

Top Anti-Ageing Tips

- Best anti-ageing product for young people is high factor sunscreen to the face/neck/hands.

- Smoking should be avoided as this accelerates skin ageing (amongst many other adverse effects).

- Use anti-ageing topical products for at least six to 12 months to get the full benefit.

- Over the counter anti-wrinkle creams containing retinol and retinyl can help.

- For sun-damaged skin with pigmentation spots, and mild wrinkling consider a chemical peel.

- Wrinkles on the forehead and around the eyes can lessen with Botox injections.

- Fillers can temporarily help to reduce hollows and lift cheeks and fill frown lines.

- Carbon dioxide laser can be used for severe wrinkling/sun-damage pigment spots on the face.

- Intense pulsed light is good at reducing pigmentation spots on the face/hands.

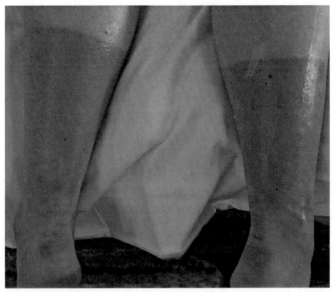

Sun burn on the back of lower legs

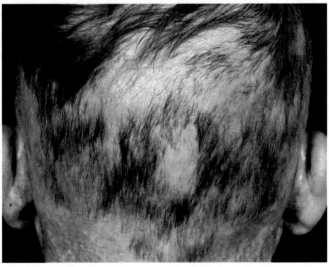

Alopecia areata patchy hairloss scalp

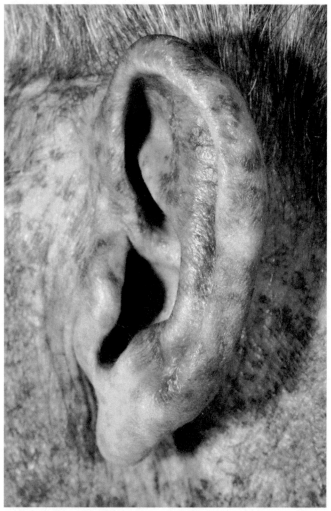

Sun damaged skin with freckling on ear

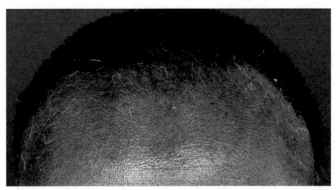

Scarring hair loss caused by frontal fibrosing alopecia

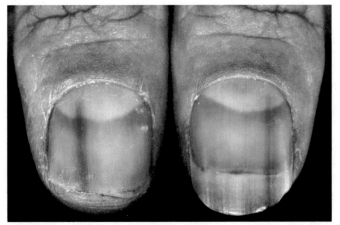

Harmless moles under nails causing linear melanonychia

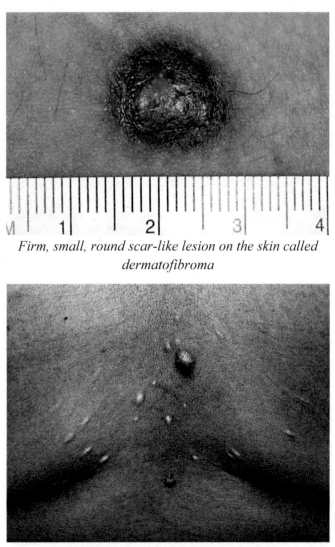

Firm, small, round scar-like lesion on the skin called dermatofibroma

Bumpy scarring on the back from chicken pox

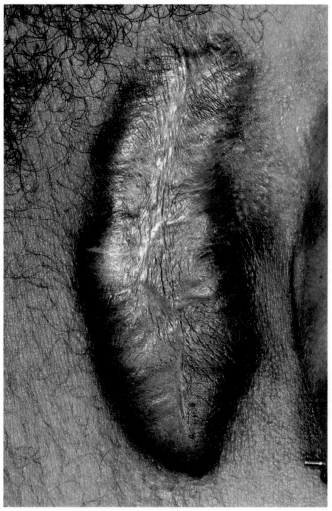

Keloid scar behind ear

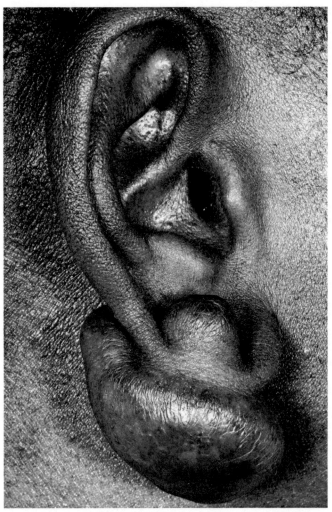

So-called dumbbell keloid scar from ear piercing

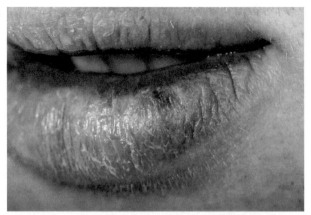

Harmless freckle on the lip called labial macule

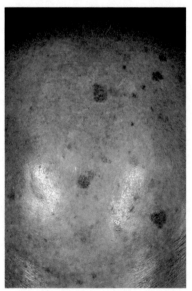

Large harmless freckles called solar lentigos on the scalp showing sun damage

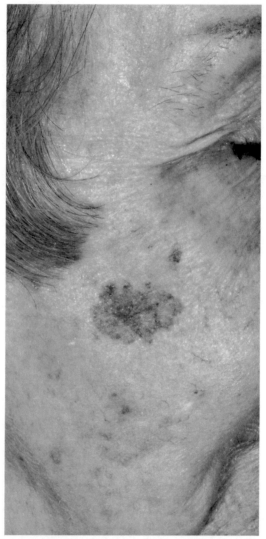

Large pigmented patch on the cheek which is a premalignant lentigo maligna

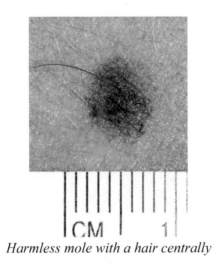

Harmless mole with a hair centrally

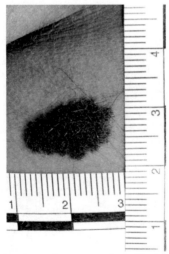

Harmless birthmark-type mole called a congenital naevus

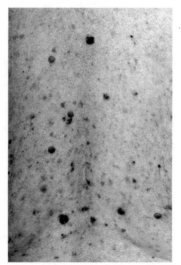

Multiple brown harmless lesions called Seborrhoeic keratoses and fleshy moles

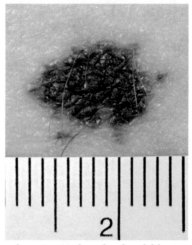

Irregular atypical mole should be excised

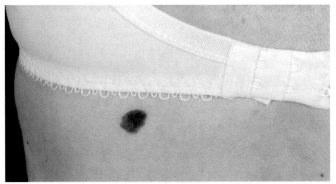

Superficial spreading melanoma

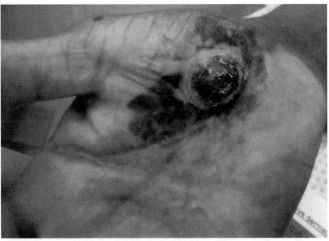

Background pigment is melanoma with a nodule within it on the palm

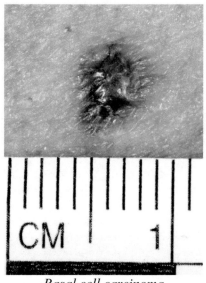

Basal cell carcinoma

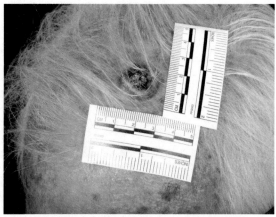

Squamous cell carcinoma of the scalp

CHAPTER 6

Moisture and the Skin

How does the skin act as a barrier? Why does your skin wrinkle when you sit for a long time in the bath? What causes atopic dermatitis (eczema)? Why does our skin get drier as we get older? Does using oil in the bath really moisturise your skin? Do statins dry our skin out?

To sustain life on dry land we need to have some sort of barrier to desiccation. It's often been said that the skin keeps our insides in and the outside world out. But is our skin really an armour-like barrier protecting us from harm? At the microscopic level, we can see that our skin is in fact is a permeable barrier constructed a bit like a modern brick wall. In the stratum corneum (outer layer of the skin) there are bricks (corneocytes) embedded in mortar (lipid-rich matrix). The bricks and mortar are stacked into bi-layers with water-repellent lipids around them. This lipid bilayer restricts water flowing out of our skin and the inward movement of toxins, allergens and germs. The lipids (ceramides and fatty acids) are made by lamellar bodies which secrete them out into the bilayer. Small amounts of water are naturally lost through the stratum corneum and is called transepidermal water loss (TEWL). So the construction and performance of this lipid bilayer is crucial to our skin barrier function.

The slightly acid pH of the skin is also very important for barrier function as we know that imbalances can lead to skin disease. Interestingly there is a lower ph. found in the axillae (arm pits), in the groin and between the toes – all sites where skin infections are more common with fungi and bacteria. Natural skin ph. is around 5, so using products that help to maintain that ph. will help moisture retention in the skin and reduce the chance of colonisation/infection of the skin.

So what happens when our skin barrier is not working properly? The insides start seeping out and noxious substances from the outside world can get in. The most common example of this is eczema, which affects 3.5% of the global population. Eczema (synonymous with dermatitis) comes from the Greek word meaning 'to boil'. There are lots of different types of eczema that can affect us at any age, but probably the best-known form is the one that starts in young children called atopic eczema (atopic dermatitis). A mutation in the filaggrin gene which is partly responsible for controlling the lipid secretion is thought to be the cause of the malfunctioning lipid bilayer. This loss of barrier function means the skin dries out (increased TEWL) and bacteria can get in. Eczema sufferers have dry, red flaky skin that is very itchy. Scratching is almost inevitable because the itching can be very severe, leading to further breakdown of the skin surface. Bacteria called *Staphylococcus aureus* tend to move into the broken inflamed skin, causing localised infection. Soon a vicious cycle is set up of inflammation and infection, itching and scratching.

The 'leaky' barrier function can also allow in small protein particles and chemicals that are then recognised as 'foreign' material by the skin, leading to the development of allergies. So if you suffer from eczema then you are more likely to develop an allergy to products coming into contact with your skin than those with a normal barrier function. These contact allergies usually develop through chronic repeated exposure to the same products/substances (allergen) over and over again. Common contact allergens include perfumes (parfum on the product label), chemical preservatives (used to stop products 'going-off') and nickel (a metal used in jewellery/clothing/mobile phones). Reactions appear within a few days of contact with the allergen and look like patches of eczema. So having an eczema tendency can lead to the development of allergic contact dermatitis which appears as a patch of eczema!

Babies and young infants with atopic eczema can develop food allergies and the current evidence suggests they are sensitized to the foods (become allergic to them) through their inflamed eczema skin, and not through their gut. In other words, if babies/young infants eat peanuts (in the form of smooth peanut butter) egg, wheat, soya, cow's milk, fish etc at an early age (from 6 months) they are less likely to become allergic to these foods than if they are exposed to small amounts of the food proteins just through their skin.

This is a complete paradigm shift from the advice given to parents just a few years ago, when they were told to avoid giving young babies with atopic eczema nuts, cow's milk etc. However, in actual fact, this led to the development of more, not less food allergies.

We can now see why the treatment of eczema aims to restore the vital barrier function, by rehydrating the skin, replacing lipids and reducing inflammation. Emollients (moisturisers) are the mainstay of treatment for all dry skin conditions including eczema and psoriasis. The Holy Grail however of eczema research over the past two decades has been to try to find a way of permanently restoring the barrier function. Ultimately for those suffering from atopic eczema, 'gene therapy' may be available. Correction of the filaggrin gene mutation in the form of cream that is rubbed onto the affected skin, might sound like something out of a sci-fi movie, but the reality is, this may not be that far away.

So what about other common causes of dry skin? As we get older our skin becomes drier, especially on our hands and lower legs. So what is happening in our skin to cause this? The process of natural intrinsic ageing in the skin seems to start from the age 20 years onwards. After this we produce 1% less collagen each year (that's a big loss of production when you get to my age!). The surface cells (keratinocytes) tend to accumulate in clumps on the skin surface leading to the appearance of dry flakes. The fat cells underneath start to shrink a bit and this leads to a reduction in water transfer into the upper skin layers. Finally from age 50 onwards the sebaceous (oil) glands start to shrink, leading to less oil in the skin. The areas of our skin with the smallest number of sebaceous glands are the most susceptible to this drying effect, namely the lower legs and hands.

So as we get older we want to try to preserve lipid in our skin and keep it out of our circulation. Many people over the age of 50 currently take a statin medication prescribed by their doctor to lower their blood cholesterol and triglyceride levels (fats in the blood). It was thought initially that these medicines also reduced the level of lipid/cholesterol in the skin, causing additional drying effects. However most studies now agree that these effects in the skin are minimal, with only occasional drying of the lips (chelitis) being a problem. Some statins have recently even been shown to be therapeutically beneficial in treating a dry skin condition called psoriasis.

To try to combat dry skin conditions, moisturisers (emollients) have been used for hundreds of years. But how do moisturisers actually work? Do they get moisture into the skin or do they stop us losing moisture? In fact the answer is both, depending on what the constituents of the moisturiser are. There are two main types of ingredients in an emollient: humectants (water holding) which attract water from the depths of the skin (such as urea, propylene glycol, glycerine and hydroxyl acids) and occlusive (paraffin, lanolin, mineral oils) that create an oily barrier at the skin surface, sealing in water and reducing evaporation. Paraffin for example is known to block water loss by penetrating into the spaces between the cells in the skin. Mixtures of lipids have been shown to accelerate the restoration of barrier function and therefore the most effective moisturisers contain both humectants and occlusive.

Emollient properties:

- Treat dry/scaly/inflamed skin.
- Reduce transepidermal water loss (TEWL).
- Increase barrier function.
- Soften dry skin.
- Ease itching.
- Reduce scaling.
- Allow active ingredients into the skin.

People who have normal skin don't need to use moisturisers. Their skin is in its own natural balance and doesn't need adjusting. Those of us with an oily skin may find that our skin is also dry (so-called combination), because we are lacking water in our skin, so we should use light watery moisturisers to help redress the balance. Those of us with a dry/flaky skin may need a much richer oily emollient, but with some watery component in it. In addition, different parts of our skin need different types of emollients. Generally, it is recommended we avoid heavy oily emollients on our face where clogging pores can lead to acne. Lower legs and feet/hands are generally much drier than the rest of our skin and rich oily emollients are needed.

Emollient formulation	Properties
Ointment	Oil based, occlusive, less preservatives needed, rich hydration
Cream	Emulsion of oil/water, contain chemical preservatives, medium hydration
Lotion	Watery suspensions, may contain alcohol, easy to spread over large areas, lower hydration
Gel	Semisolid emulsion, usually in alcohol, well absorbed, dries on the skin, minimal hydration

There has been a lot of controversy in the medical literature about whether or not bath oils help to moisturise the skin. Can adding an emollient to the water help to stop our skin drying out? It seems strange to think that water can be drying to the skin. So how is that possible, and why does our skin wrinkle when we have been sitting in the bath for a long time? Our standard understanding is that water enters the skin from the bath-water by osmosis. This water saturates the stratum corneum, making it expand, as all the cells swell. The top layer of the skin enlarges so much that it starts to form ridges or wrinkles on the skin surface. So far so good. But then why doesn't all our skin wrinkle in the bath, why only our hands and feet? We have always thought this was due to the fact that the skin on our hands and feet is the thickest and therefore can swell the most.

However, recent experiments have shown that if the sympathetic (autonomic, flight/fright) nerve is cut, then no wrinkling occurs on water-immersion. It is therefore thought that the water coming in by osmosis stimulates the sympathetic nerve to fire off, leading to blood vessel shut-down (vasoconstriction), which then actually leads to loss of volume, negative pressure and pulling down of the overlying skin into wrinkles. So the skin is in fact drying out and not becoming hydrated with water. Nonetheless it remains a hotly debated topic amongst scientists, and whatever the underlying mechanism, you will notice that having wrinkled fingers increases your grip in water, which is handy when you're doing the washing up!

So back to the bath oil. Can moisturising bath products help to combat the drying effect of water, particularly for those suffering from dry skin? A study in newborns found that in the first few days of life, using bath oil seemed to impair maturation of the skin barrier function by actually increasing TEWL. However, another very interesting study in Norway recruited 56 six-week-old infants at their routine baby check, who were noted to have dry skin, but not eczema. Half were issued bath oil to be used five to seven times per week plus a rich moisturising cream and the other half were not given any instructions and were just observed. Babies were assessed again at three and six months. At six months follow-up, there were statistically significantly different results between the two groups. In the moisturising group 75% of the babies had normal skin versus 37% in the observation group. In addition, in the observation group 19% of the babies now had obvious atopic eczema as opposed to only 4% in the moisturising group. So good evidence that if your baby has dry skin by the age six weeks they do benefit from bath oil and emollient, and this may even prevent the onset of atopic eczema in the first few months of life.

Properties of Soap Substitutes

- Cleansing cream formulations, therefore hydrating not drying.

- Remove grease/dirt from the skin, cleaning without 'bubbles'.

- Some contain disinfectant to kill bacteria (*E. coli* and MRSA).

- Generally don't contain surfactant, therefore less irritant to dry skin.

It does seem overall that we can rehydrate our skin with moisturising preparations. But which one to choose when you are bombarded by an array of multiple products on the shelves, can be difficult. As a general rule most dermatologists don't think that aqueous cream or plain oil by themselves are good moisturisers. Aqueous cream as the name suggests is very watery so it seeps in very well but quickly evaporates and is therefore not highly hydrating. Oil on the other hand such as olive oil or nut oil can sit on the skin surface and not penetrate very well to aid deep hydration. However, if you mixed those two components together you would get an emulsion that was full of lipid and water, a good balanced emollient. Manufacturers try to formulate their moisturising creams with a good balance between water and lipid, with a different ratio of each to produce either 'light' or 'rich' emollients. They try to avoid the most irritant/sensitizing preservatives, irritant surfactants and alkaline chemicals that might destabilise the skin's ph.

So if you decide your skin is dry and you need to buy a moisturiser then think about which part of your skin is dry and choose an emollient suitable for that site. If it's just your face then choose smaller volume pots with extra hydration for around the eyes and then a light, more watery cream for the rest of the face. If you have dry lips, then use lipsalve regularly during the day and thick plain Vaseline at night.

Hand creams are usually very hydrating but non-greasy so you can still use your hands after the cream is applied. You could consider applying the cream to your hands in a generous amount at night and then putting cotton gloves over the top. This occlusion by the cotton gloves helps to drive the cream into the dry skin overnight, making moisturising much more effective. The lower legs can often be very dry, so here you should choose a large tub of thick/rich oily emollient to allow you to apply generous amounts several times each day. Emollient creams containing 10% urea are very effective at softening and smoothing very thick rough skin. The main thing is to find a moisturiser that you actually like as you will be much more inclined to use it regularly.

Top Moisturising Tips

- Only use moisturisers if your skin is dry or needs hydrating.

- If your baby has dry skin use regular emollients.

- Choose moisturisers suitable for the site of dry skin.

- Avoid heavy oily emollients on the face, except round the eyes.

- Apply moisturiser under cotton gloves to dry hands overnight.

- Lotions are good for application to hair-bearing sites.

- Soap substitutes can help reduce drying and irritating effects of soap bars on dry skin.

- Find a moisturiser you like and then use it regularly.

CHAPTER 7

*Hair Growth, What Causes our Hair to
Grow/Fall Out?*

*What do we really understand about our hair? How does
it grow? Why do we lose hair on the tops of our head as
we age but keep the hair at the back? Why does our hair
turn grey as we get older?*

The study of hair is a fascinating and challenging area of
science. We have come a long way in our understanding
about what causes hair to grow and fall out. But it's fair
to say that we frequently don't have very effective or
lasting solutions to the problems we experience with our
hair. It may be tempting to wish for something we don't
have, such as those with wavy hair wishing it was
straight, those with straight hair wishing it was wavy.
We may want more hair on our scalp and less hair
elsewhere on our bodies. We often have an idea of how
we think our hair should look and we may spend lots of
time and money trying to achieve this.

To try to answer some of the questions that are frequently asked about hair, we first need to understand a little bit about how hair grows and what influences that. When we are born, we have about five million hairs and we won't gain any more as we grow older, we will only lose hairs. We have hairs on all of our skin except the palms and soles.

There are differences in our hair associated with our genetics and ethnicity. For example, Asians have thick hair strands which are usually straight with a density of 90,000 follicles on the scalp. Caucasians by contrast have 120,000 hair follicles on their scalp, but the diameter of the hairs is less thick than Asians, and they can have hair that is wavy/straight or curly. Those of African descent have 90,000 scalp follicles, their hair is usually curly, and each hair is thinner in diameter, then Caucasian and Asian hair.

So Asians have the thickest hair strands and those of African descent the thinnest hair strands. Caucasians have the highest density of hair follicles on the scalp. So how do we account for these structural differences?

The hair strand itself is made up of proteins and chemicals and consists of three layers: an inner cortex, outer cuticle and medulla in the middle. The medulla is absent in fine hair of children. The outer cuticle consists of overlapping keratin scales (a bit like roof tiles) which protect the delicate hair structure underneath. Asians hair cuticle is made up over six to eight scales thick, slightly less in Caucasians and even less in those with African hair. Having a thinner cuticle means African hair is more prone to breakage. When our hair is wet the proteins can be reversibly stretched by up to 30%, but above that we risk permanent damage and ultimately hair fracture.

Natural curling of the hair occurs due to variation in diameter along the hair shaft, the diameter at twisting points is smaller than the straight areas, and it has an ellipse shape in cross-section. Straight Asian hair by contrast has an equal diameter along the whole hair shaft which is cylindrical in cross-section.

In addition, the hair at each body site is quite different and distinctive in its characteristics. For example eyelash hair doesn't grow very long when you compare it to scalp hair, and hair on our arms tends to be much finer than hair in the pubic or armpit regions.

Like plants, hairs have roots from which they grow. The hair follicle grows from the hair root which is located in the dermis of the skin. The root feeds the hair with blood and nutrients and as it grows it pushes the hair out from the skin surface. As it passes through the opening a small amount of oil (from the sebaceous glands) is coated onto the hair to lubricate it. Hair strands at the surface are dead (that's why having our hair cut is not painful). The live hair root is the hair's 'command centre' where control over the hair characteristics is determined, such as hair length, its colour, its diameter and whether it is wavy or straight. Your age and sex can also affect how hair grows. For example men's hair grows faster than women's hair. Asians have a longer hair growing phase than Caucasians and can therefore grow their hair longer.

The plant analogy is a useful one, as just like the leaves on deciduous trees, hairs have a growing phase, resting phase and shedding phase. However, unlike some trees which shed all their leaves simultaneously, we don't 'moult', as all of our hairs are simultaneously in different phases of the hair cycle. The length of these phases and how many hairs are in each phase at any one time will determine the length and density of our hair.

We have about 100,000 hair follicles on our scalp and about 85% of these will be in a growing phase (anergen) at any one time. On average our scalp hair grows 15cm per year (faster in the summer than the winter) and anergen can last between two and six years, so you can, if you wish, grow your scalp hair quite long (15cm x 6 years = 90cm). Contrast that with eyelash hairs where about 30% of the hairs are in anergen at any one time and it lasts only about seven weeks. So we can see why we don't usually need to trim our eyelashes.

1% of the hair follicles at any one time are instructed by the body to stop growing (catergen phase), and during this 10-14 day period the follicle shrinks back. Hair then enters the final and third stage of the hair cycle which is the shedding (telogen phase). Approximately 10-15% of scalp hairs are in a telogen phase at any given time, which translates into 50-100 scalp hairs being shed every day. After the hair is shed the follicle then rests for up to four months before starting to grow again. Usually each hair is at a different stage of the hair cycle so that all our hair doesn't fall out at once. However in certain situations this can happen.

A large number of our hairs can be induced into a shedding phase all at once, so-called, telogen effluviam (which is diffuse hair shedding leading to loss of hair density). This can occur six-12 weeks after a 'stressful' event in the body such as giving birth, some types of chemotherapy (where up to 50% of the hair is shed), being seriously ill, having a high fever, weight loss on a low calorie/restrictive diet and sustaining major psychological stress. The good news is that telogen effluvium usually recovers after six months and then the hair should start to recover. However if the events that caused it are repeated then normal hair growth may be very fragmented.

Some types of chemotherapy can cause rapid and complete hair loss, as the drugs target any rapidly dividing cells in the body, which includes the hair follicles. This is called anergen effluvium and can be a very distressing side effect of the cancer treatment for both women and men. Hair starts to fall out within two to four weeks of commencing the treatment and may take months to recover, once the chemotherapy has finished. Curiously, when the hair starts to grow back it may be a slightly different colour and texture from your previous hair.

Oncologists have tried various strategies to try to prevent/minimise scalp hair loss associated with chemotherapy, by for example, cooling the scalp. A group in the Netherlands recently published a study that compared 160 patients (scalp-cooled) with 86 patients (non-scalp cooled) who were undergoing chemotherapy for several types of cancer. Overall the use of wigs/scalp coverings was reduced by 40% in the scalp cooled group. So definitely a modest benefit was demonstrated in this study by cooling the scalp just prior to administering chemotherapy.

Other causes of hair loss include an autoimmune condition called alopecia areata (AA). In this condition your own white cells (lymphocytes) start attacking your own hair follicles, causing the hair to fall out diffusely or more commonly, in circular patches. It can be very alarming as it may literally occur over a few days or weeks without any obvious trigger. It's a common condition estimated to affect about 2% of people at some point in their lives. Thankfully the majority of people affected do recover their hair growth spontaneously, but the condition can wax and wane over time. When the hair starts to grow back it is white at first before the previous hair colour returns. Some patients can have very extensive alopecia areata and they can lose all their scalp hair and even eyelashes/eyebrows too, which can be very distressing. Thankfully this type of AA is relatively rare.

Much more common, however, is the main cause of hair loss worldwide, which is 'natural hair loss' that affects about 50% of males and about 40% of post-menopausal females. Some people refer to this type of progressive permanent hair thinning of the scalp as 'male-pattern hair loss' or just 'pattern hair loss' (as females and makes are affected); but perhaps the best term is androgenetic alopecia. So what is it that causes about half the population to lose their hair as they get older?

The short answer is genetics. Large studies have identified two main genes linked to androgenetic alopecia, one on chromosome 20 (20p11) and one on the X chromosome. Men only have one X-chromosome and they get this from their mother. This X could have been passed on to her by her father or her mother. So looking at your maternal grandfather's hair is no guarantee of balding or keeping a full head of hair yourself in the future. The alopecia gene found on chromosome 20 is estimated to increase the risk of balding by three to four times, so the X-chromosome is by no means the main determinant of hair loss or retention. It is estimated overall that 80% of balding is genetic and the other 20% is accounted for by factors such as stress, chronic illness, hormone imbalances, medications, iron levels etc.

In androgenetic alopecia there is increased hair shedding and each hair's diameter becomes narrower, leading to fine downy-type (vellus) hair on the scalp, called miniaturisation. In the early stages in men there is classically frontal recession in the temple regions and then loss of hair at the crown (scalp vertex). In women the frontal hairline is usually preserved, however they develop hair miniaturisation at the vertex.

Each hair on the scalp carries genetic information that determines whether and when that hair might develop sensitivity to androgens, and therefore shedding/miniaturisation. The most important of these is being sensitive to dihydrotestosterone (DHT). Once a hair becomes sensitive to DHT then the miniaturisation process starts. Interestingly, hairs at the back of the scalp (the occipital region) do not develop sensitivity to DHT and therefore remain, long after all the other scalp hairs have gone. This is the reason why these occipital hairs are used in hair transplants.

The hair transplant surgeon excises a strip of skin from the posterior occipital scalp and dissects out the hairs into 'mini-grafts' which are transplanted into slits made in the frontal scalp skin. The occipital hairs retain their protection from DHT even when transplanted, so the hairs don't fall out or miniaturise. Depending on the extent of the baldness, three to five graft sessions are required over one to two years to regain the desired 'full head of hair'. So ultimately if we could stop all of our scalp hair from being sensitive to DHT in the first place, then we could potentially eliminate premature balding.

Eyebrow restoration by hair transplantation has also recently been shown to be effective for those who have permanently lost eyebrow hairs through trauma, surgery or inflammatory skin diseases. Hair grafts are again harvested from the occipital scalp and transplanted into the eyebrow area. Results are very promising, but because occipital hair grows faster than normal eyebrow hairs, the transplanted hairs need to be trimmed regularly to maintain an even appearance.

Another interesting way to try to stimulate eyelash/eyebrow hair to grow is by using some eye drops that were originally designed to treat glaucoma (which is a condition where there is raised pressure in the eye).

When glaucoma patients were treated with bimatoprost eye drops, doctors noticed that as a side effect the patient's eyelashes grew longer and thicker. So a product called Latisse was manufactured (FDA approval in 2008) to help improve eyelash growth. Latisse should only be applied to the upper eyelid (never dropped into the eye) and with blinking will automatically be transferred to the lower lid margins. This has been used by doctors to help restore eyelash and eyebrow hair in patients suffering from AA.

Latisse seems to be lengthening the hair's growing phase and increasing hair density. It can even cause the hair to become darker. One potential (and apparently rare side effect) is permanent eye colour change; so in other words if you have blue eyes, they could permanently change to brown with use of this product. It is very expensive, $120 for a one-month supply, and has been used by some celebrities. Sadly, Lattise doesn't seem to work on scalp hair, but the science is very interesting and with more investigation perhaps we can use this knowledge to come up with something that does work for scalp hair in the future.

Conventionally those trying to reverse the miniaturisation process have turned to the use of topical, or oral minoxidil (Rogaine/Regaine). Oral minoxidil was initially used as an antihypertensive medication (lowers raised blood pressure), but doctors noticed those taking it developed increased hair growth. This observation led to the development of a 2% topical solution of minoxidil to be applied to the balding scalp.

In studies 40% of men who used topical 2% minoxidil for three to six months benefitted from moderate hair regrowth at the crown. Minoxidil lengthens the anergen phase and shortens the telogen phase of the hair cycle. Modern formulations include a 5% foam which should be applied to the affected area of the scalp twice daily for men and once daily for women. This treatment has to be continued daily for the benefits to last. Stopping the minoxidil allows the effects of dihydrotestosterone to start the miniaturisation process again.

Oral finasteride (propecia) works by reducing dihydrotestosterone levels around the hair follicles by 70% and therefore reduces progressive miniaturisation. Dutasteride is a more potent blocker of DHT than finasteride, leading to 90% reduction in DHT levels. Both oral treatments can be safely taken by men and post-menopausal women. In studies 80% of those taking finasteride/dutasteride had significantly increased hair density and hair shaft diameter on the scalp after one year. However, just like minoxidil these medications need to be taken daily and must be continued for as long as the effect on the hair follicles is desired. Stopping these medicines leads to all the beneficial effects being reversed after six months.

New topical formulations combining minoxidil and finasteride have recently been launched as a hair density maintenance treatment after taking oral finasteride or dutasteride for two years. This helps those who are bothered by the side effects of finasteride (low libido, erectile dysfunction, enlarged breast tissue) to switch to topical therapy which generally has less side effects.

Treatment for androgenetic alopecia is not available free on the NHS in the UK. Topical minoxidil can be bought over the counter at the chemist and oral finasteride/dutasteride is only available by paying for private prescriptions.

Not only does our hair shed and miniaturise as we get older it can also turn a white colour (called achromotrichia). The term 'grey hair' is actually a misnomer: hair in fact turns white, not grey. When we see 'grey hair' what we are actually observing is the overall appearance when the white and the dark hairs occur together. Generally speaking, hair turns white first on the scalp, then the beard area, then the body and finally the eyebrows. Hair specialists often refer to the '50-50-50 rule' which says that in the general population, by the age of 50 years, 50% of us will be 50% 'grey'.

So why is that? And what causes our hair to be brown, black, blond or red in the first place?

Down at the hair bulb our hair colour is determined by the amount and type of melanin pigment present. There are two main types of melanin: eumelanin (brown, black) and phaeomelanin (blond/red). Your genetic makeup helps determine which type of melanin your body predominantly produces. For example those with red hair only produce phaeomelanin. People with blond hair produce small amounts of eumelanin, and those with brown hair produce medium amounts of eumelanin. Those individuals with very shiny black hair produce lots of eumelanin (which gives the hair the black colour) but they also produce very small amounts of pheomelanin (which gives the hair the appearance of shine).

Melanocytes (pigment producing cells) inside the hair follicles produce the melanin (using an enzyme called tyrosinase), which is deposited in the cortex (the middle section) of the hair shaft and gives the hair its colour. Interestingly the melanocytes in the eyebrow hairs are usually more active than at other hair sites, leading to darker hair at the eyebrows than elsewhere on the body. The activity of the melanocytes can also change with age. Many blond children develop darker brown hair as they get older as their melanocytes become more active and produce more of the eumelanin pigment.

As we age our melanocyte stem cells start to die, and with less melanocytes around there is a reduction in melanin production. In addition, as we get older we have less of the enzyme tyrosinase, which is needed to synthesize melanin. The hair shaft is therefore given less and less melanin pigment and eventually all we see is the colour of keratin sheath, which is white. There is also a build-up of hydrogen peroxide (bleach) around the hair shaft due to lower levels of the catalase enzyme needed to break down hydrogen peroxide. So a combination of these processes lead to loss of our natural hair colour.

Surveys have shown that people associate the colour grey with drab, dingy, conformity and not surprisingly, old age. However, having grey or white hair can convey a sense of gravitas, seniority, chic, sophistication and attractiveness. So called 'salt and pepper' hair is currently a popular trend in the fashion industry with 'salt' being silver and 'pepper' being grey. Many famous icons have 'gone grey gracefully', such as George Clooney, Barack Obama, Jamie Lee Curtis and Renee Davis. So having grey hair can be hugely enhancing. This current opinion is neatly demonstrated by an 80% increase in sales of grey/silver hair dye on Amazon alone.

You may have observed yourself that Caucasians' hair turns grey at a younger age than Asians', who turn grey at a younger age than Africans. So again it is likely that genetic factors play a dominant role in the age and speed of onset of greying. However other factors that might also play a role include lifestyle factors such as stress, smoking, poor diet and medical conditions such as anaemia and thyroid imbalances.

One example of very premature whitening of the hair is seen in Werner's syndrome (adult progeria), which is a genetic disorder that causes premature ageing of the body. Those affected develop premature ageing of their internal organs alongside premature whitening of their hair.

What about more common causes for premature white hair? You will sometimes hear people saying that stress has 'turned their hair grey', but is that really possible, or is it another myth? In 2012 the Nobel Prize winner in chemistry, Robert Lefkowitz showed for the first time that it was indeed true, that stress can turn our hair white.

Lefkowitz showed that stress causes a release of fight/flight neurotransmitters (nerve signals), and whilst that can be hugely helpful for preparing our body to run away from danger or fight off attackers, over long periods of time regular release of these fight/flight neurotransmitters causes damage to our DNA, which promotes ageing. These ageing effects associated with stress include tumour production, miscarriages, psychiatric disorders and whitening of the hair. So yet more reasons to try to reduce stress in our lives.

Smoking turns our hair white and promotes premature androgenetic alopecia. It is thought that the smoke affects the small blood vessels in the skin, leading to DNA damage in the hair follicles. This accelerates the process of miniaturisation and switching off melanin production. In addition, once a smoker's hair is white they are vulnerable to their hair turning an orange colour due to nicotine staining from the smoke. This orange nicotine staining is common on the skin of the fingers that hold the cigarette but can also affect white scalp/moustache hair.

Aside from the cosmetic appearance of white hair, a recent study published by a team in Turkey also showed that white hair may be a marker for underlying disease. They found that in men the degree of coronary artery disease that they were suffering from correlated with how much white scalp hair they had. This was an independent risk factor not related to their age. So early whitening of the hair could be a sign of premature biological ageing.

In general terms, once hair starts to turn white the process is usually slowly progressive. However, there have been reports of this biological 'hair clock' being reversed. Sporadic cases written up in the medical literature report some women with breast cancer treated with tamoxifen (a selective oestrogen receptor modulator mediation) who noticed that their white hair re-pigmented. Recent studies exploring this phenomenon showed that tamoxifen does indeed up-regulate melanin production by melanocytes in the laboratory. In addition, a powerful drug used to treat certain types of leukaemia (blood cancer), called Imatinib (Gleevec) has been shown to reverse the hair whitening process. So it may be possible to use this knowledge of specific chemical interactions to reverse the whitening process in the future, if we so wish.

Top Hair Facts

- Genetics controls our hair growth, density and natural hair state.

- Hair growth is adversely affected by smoking, low iron levels and calorie restricted diets.

- About 50% of us will 'thin on top' by the time we are 50 years of age.

- Dramatic hair shedding (telogen effluvium) can occur six to 12 weeks after a stressful event.

- Androgenetic alopecia in men and women can be treated with 5% topical minoxidil.

- Oral finasteride or dutasteride can treat androgenetic alopecia in men and post-menopausal women.

- Premature whitening of our hair can be caused by stress.

- Our eyebrow hair usually turns white last.

- Cardiovascular disease is associated with premature hair whitening.

- Sales of grey/silver hair dye have increased by 80% over the last few years.

CHAPTER 8

Hair Care and Styling

What does shampoo and conditioner actually do? How does hair styling work? Does blow drying damage our hair? What does straightening and relaxing do to hair structure? What are the chemicals in hair dye? Can hair treatments actually cause our hair to fall out? What causes dandruff and can I get rid of it?

There is evidence from Egyptian mummies that we have been 'enhancing' our hair for thousands of years, so what we do today is really nothing new. Analysis of mummies has shown that the Egyptians used a 'fat-based' hair gel to mould and hold their hair into position. They also used hair dye, hair braiding, wigs, hair extensions and even curling tongs have been found inside some tombs.

Globally, the majority of the population may not do very much with their scalp hair, but there is evidence that the most will brush or comb their hair at some point and use shampoo/conditioner from time to time. So, what does brushing and the use of products do to enhance our 'dead hair shafts'?

Brushing our hair separates the hair strands from each other, causing the hair to look smoother and therefore shinier. Nonetheless, vigorous hair brushing (I do remember as a child my mother fighting with knots in my tangled hair) can irritate the scalp skin and may pull out hairs prematurely that weren't ready to be shed. Vigorous hair combing/brushing can cause inflammation around the hair bulb and if this becomes chronic, may lead to permanent damage to some of the hair follicles. So generally speaking, gentle limited brushing is probably better than the '100 strokes' that was recommended to me as a child to ensure I had knot-free hair.

Most of us use shampoo to wash our scalp skin/hair, but why do we use it, and what frequency is recommended? If we used plain water to wash our hair then it would be difficult to extract dirt and sebum (naturally occurring skin oil) from it. You might be surprised to hear that shampoos can contain up to 30 different chemical ingredients, so they are certainly not all the same. However, they all contain detergents (surfactants) which can attract water and oil to themselves and lower surface tension. This allows mixing of water/oil and other agents such as emulsifiers, keratins and perfumes, which then clean and refresh our scalp skin and hair.

Washing our hair daily with detergents can remove too much of the natural oil (sebum), and this results in our hair becoming dry and brittle. Dry hair tends to stick together, leading to knots. In fact, washing hair daily removes the sebum so efficiently that is prompts the scalp to produce more, setting up a 'vicious cycle' of washing to remove oil and then increased oil production. This stripping of our natural sebum has led some people to advocate leaving our hair to 'wash itself', rather than using chemical shampoos. Generally speaking washing hair every two to three days is probably the healthiest frequency, nonetheless many of us wash our hair daily.

What about anti-dandruff shampoos? Do they really work? Well, to answer that question we really need to know what dandruff is. When we think of dandruff we think of flaking, usually in the scalp. Flakes drop off and we sometimes see them on our clothes. There are a number of causes of these flakes, including dry skin conditions such as eczema and psoriasis; insufficient shampooing which leads to a build-up of skin cells/oils on the scalp; sensitivity to hair care products such as preservatives in shampoos, leading to allergic of irritant contact dermatitis.

However, one of the main causes of dandruff appears to be caused by a sensitivity to a yeast that is found on our skin in oil (sebum) rich areas such as the scalp, face and anterior chest. The yeast is called *Malassezia globosa* and it is naturally found on our skin, it grows well in oily conditions. This yeast overgrowth in some people stimulates an immune reaction, possibly as a result of a reaction to enzymes called lipase that the yeast produces to help break down sebum.

The result is slightly red and inflamed skin, which turns over more quickly causing scaling and ultimately flakes to appear at the affected skin sites. So most anti-dandruff shampoos are designed to help lift out the flakes and they should also help to kill/inhibit the yeast. However, if you stop using the anti-dandruff shampoo then the condition returns, as the yeast is part of our natural skin flora and always comes back.

So to keep on top of the problem you need to continue using the anti-dandruff shampoo two to three times per week. Sometimes medical practitioners prescribe topical steroids to help reduce the itching and inflammation that can occur when the seborrheic dermatitis is very active, and this helps to switch off the reaction. If the condition is very severe then sometimes a short course of itraconazole anti-fungal tablets are prescribed to help kill the yeast and get things back under control before maintenance anti-fungal shampoo can start working again.

So combatting dry itchy scalps can be a challenge and often requires ongoing attention. However, the hair itself can also become very dry and may need moisturising with so-called 'conditioners'. What they do is to try to combat stripping of the natural oils that are leached out of the hair during washing. Conditioners usually contain silicones and fatty acids that coat the hairs and stop them sticking together. Custom formulated conditioners contain molecules that are 'positively charged' which makes the hair strands 'repel' each other, leading to a smoothing non-tangled effect.

2-in-1 shampoos have a 'conditioning' component to them such as silicone/fatty acids in addition to the detergent, but these are generally 'non-charged'. As the product is rinsed off the hair the conditioner binds to the hair shafts as the detergent washes away. So 2-in-1 products are very convenient but some argue that are not as intensely conditioning as stand-alone products, although they have come a long way since the initial 'Wash and Go' products. Naturally dry and colour treated hair, which also has a tendency to dryness, usually benefits from a conditioner with a high concentration of silicone.

So shampoo and conditioner are not really altering our 'dead hair cuticles' but they do remove dirt and make the surface smooth, shiny, more manageable and less full of static cling ('fly away'). After washing and conditioning some people leave their hair to dry naturally. To facilitate this some will use a towel to rub their hair dry: however, there is evidence that vigorous rubbing damages the hair cuticle, causing it to flake. Blotting drying hair is the recommended method over rubbing dry to prevent damaging it.

Using a hair dryer (blow-dryer) is a fast-reliable way to dry hair. Heat accelerates water evaporation from the hair and creates temporary hydrogen bonds within the hair strands which facilitate shaping and styling (hold, lift and volume). These hydrogen bonds are actually quite strong; however, they are broken down readily by humidity (go out on a damp day and all that hard work styling our hair can be lost in minutes) and hair washing.

Some modern hairdryers have a 'cold shot' button which allows air at room temperature to be blown onto the hair helping to 'set' the style. Ionic technology has also been incorporated into some modern dryers which reduces static electricity build up in the hair as its drying.

Modern hairdryers can be very powerful, with outputs ranging from 900-2,300 watts, so holding them too close to the skin can lead to burning and hair cuticle damage. A Danish medical journal article published in 2014 reported parents using a hairdryer to dry their baby's buttocks. The baby had napkin rash and so the parents were trying to avoid towel drying the skin. Unfortunately, the baby's buttocks sustained a skin burn because the parents hadn't realised how powerful and hot the air was coming out of the hairdryer.

Some diabetic patients have loss of sensation in their toes due to nerve damage, which means they may be unaware of pain, and therefore more vulnerable to damage. This is illustrated by reports of diabetics using a hairdryer to dry their feet/foot casts leading to skin burns. To reduce the risk of burns with these powerful hairdryers a 'diffuser' attachment can be used. This disperses the hot air over a larger area, leading to lower contact temperature, slower drying and less physical damage to the skin/hair.

Dyson have recently launched their first hairdryer after spending £50m on research and development. The stylish hand piece is half the weight of regular hair dryers and will not exceed 150 degrees centigrade (therefore lower risk of damaging the hair cuticle and burning your ears). However, the main claim is that it dries hair eight times faster than regular hairdryers and leaves you with a smooth sleek finish. A bit of a 'game changer' according to some of those now using it, but at around £300 it will be out of most people's price range.

So blow-drying our hair leads to rapid drying and can give us a temporary style. More permanent hair styling aimed at delivering waves/curls is achieved through 'perms'. These are chemicals that break down and reform the disulphide bonds within the hair. These disulphide bonds are very strong indeed and after perming, the effects on the treated hair last about eight to 12 months, which contrasts with the hydrogen bonds formed during hot styling which last a day or two. Modern perms are much subtler than the tight curls we saw in the 1980s, and are starting to come back into fashion.

Conversely, those with naturally wavy/curly tresses may at times like to achieve a straighter hair style. Temporary solutions include the use intense heat in the form of hot tongs/flat irons. Hair is usually straightened by putting a section of hair between the two hot flat surfaces and slowly moving the tongs down the hair from the crown to the ends. This intense heat treatment can temporarily or even permanently straighten hair, depending on the temperature and number of heat cycles.

A scientific study conducted in 2013 showed that flat irons expose hair to temperatures ranging from 120-175^0C. The higher the temperatures and the higher the number of repeated heat exposures, the more likely it was that the hair would be permanently straightened. It also showed that the straightening resulted from a gradual decrease in microfilament organisation inside the hair shaft, and that silicone treatment didn't significantly affect the course of the microfilament denaturation.

Because of the concerns about the potential damage caused to hair by the repeated exposure to intense heat other methods of hair straightening were sought. These alternatives use chemicals to straighten hair, called 'relaxing'. Traditionally 1-10% sodium hydroxide, lithium hydroxide and calcium hydroxide have been used (lye-relaxers). These are alkaline (pH 9-13) chemical straighteners.

The chemicals cause swelling of the hair shaft, which results in the cuticle scales separating and allowing the alkaline product to penetrate into the hair cortex. This then breaks the structural disulphide bonds which hold the hair in its natural curl. Once the bonds have been broken the hair is mechanically straightened using a comb. The relaxer is then washed out with water, and the hair remains straight.

New hair growth will be curly and so ultimately to keep the straight appearance the new growth of hair will also need to be relaxed in the same way. Relaxing is usually repeated every four months. Care needs to be taken however not to relax the same hair fibres repeatedly as this can lead to hair breakage, frizzy hair, thinning/weakening and ultimately alopecia, which may be a permanent scarring form.

Because this method of hair straightening involves the use of potent and potentially damaging hair chemicals, it would be advisable to have these types of treatments in a salon rather than attempting them yourself at home.

Another method of hair straightening is the so-called 'Japanese hair straightening' which involves the use of ammonium thioglycolate (no-lye relaxer). This selectively weakens the hair's cysteine bonds and is then neutralised with hydrogen peroxide. A hot iron is usually applied during the process to straighten the hair. There is less damage to the hair protein with this method and less risk of scalp irritation.

If hair has been previously relaxed with the alkaline or thioglycolate then the alternative method cannot be used, as they are not compatible with each other. In addition, they cannot be used on previously bleached hair.

Because of this incompatibility between different hair treatments many people have started to straighten their hair using the 'Brazilian Keratin Treatment' (BKT). This method uses formaldehyde which cross-links keratin filaments, leaving hair straight and shiny. There have however been some concerns about the concentration of formaldehyde used and whether it is safe when people are exposed to it repeatedly. Formaldehyde is a potential carcinogen, according to the National Institute of Occupational Safety and Health, so those being exposed should be adequately protected.

A study conducted in South Africa in 2012 looked at the concentration of formaldehyde found in seven commercially available brands of BKT. The US Cosmetic Ingredient Review Expert Panel has set the safe recommended concentration of formaldehyde at 0.2%. Six of the seven brands of BKT tested had levels of formaldehyde from 0.96-1.4%, which is five times higher than the safe level recommended. Even more disturbing was the fact that five of the brands were labelled 'formaldehyde-free'. Some hair straightening products contain methylene glycol, which is produced when formaldehyde reacts with water, so this could be why they are referred to as 'formaldehyde-free'.

Although this South African study just shows a snapshot of what people may be being exposed to in one part of the world, there have been numerous alerts and concerns about formaldehyde exposure in salons across several countries. Salon workers who are carrying out these treatments on a daily basis may be being exposed to much higher levels of formaldehyde on their skin and in their lungs, than clients undergoing treatment just a few times a year. There is no doubt that more research and more regulation is needed to ensure that these products are safe to use.

So we can curl straight hair and straighten curly hair in a temporary or permanent manner if we so wish. But what about our hair colour, what if we want to change that? Just in the same way that styling can be temporary or permanent, so can hair colouring. Covering white hair was considered the main aim of some of the early commercial hair dyes, to try to restore the colour that was being lost. However, soon people of all ages and hair colours were looking to these products to give them something different rather than maintain their original hair colour.

Conventionally, those not wishing to 'turn grey gracefully' have used hair dye to disguise the white hair. Permanent dyes 'fix' colour into the white hair, but as the hair grows the white colour becomes visible again close to the scalp, where the new hair is being pushed out, the so-called 'roots'. So to maintain the desired effect, dyeing our hair needs to be repeated, usually every six to eight weeks.

During the dyeing process pigment molecules enter the hair shaft and then either stay close to the outside sheath (semi/demi-permanent) or penetrate into the cortex (permanent). The semi-permanent dyes usually don't affect the natural hair colour and wash out of the outer hair shaft after six to 20 shampoos. Permanent dyes penetrate right into the cortex, they lighten our natural hair pigment and coat the hair with the new colour in the dye.

Highlighting or lightening our hair is usually a straightforward process using a combination of peroxide and ammonia. However, if we want to darken our hair we need to bleach out its natural pigment first and then apply the dark colour. Permanent black/brown hair dyes frequently contain a chemical called PPD (para-phenylenediamine). This is widely used as it has useful properties such as a natural permanent colour and rarely fades with hair washing. However, during the dyeing process the PPD needs to be oxidised to develop the dark colour and it is this intermediate step that leads some individuals to develop an allergy to PPD. This allergy reaction is more likely to develop the more an individual has been exposed to PPD in the past.

So in other words, the more you dye your hair the more likely you are to develop an allergy to some of the chemicals in it. Hair dye allergy reactions can be very severe, causing swelling, redness and itching of the skin (contact eczema) of the scalp, face and beard area. You can develop PPD allergy from dye used in salons and dye bought over the counter for home use. If in doubt a 'skin test' can be carried out to check for PPD sensitivity; this test can be done at the hair salon, or you can do the test at home. If you develop PPD allergy then you should avoid hair dyes containing PPD, which tend to be the permanent dark dyes. Many temporary dyes don't contain PPD so they can be used instead.

Just a final word of warning: some temporary tattoos may also contain PPD, so if you are known to be allergic to PPD and you are thinking of having a temporary tattoo done, then do check what the ingredients are. Henna tattoos tend to have a rich brown/red pigment to them and are incredibly safe and very unlikely indeed to cause allergic reactions. The temporary tattoos that contain PPD tend to be a black colour, so this can be a useful marker if you're not sure.

Top Hair Care Tips

- Hair should be brushed/combed gently to avoid pulling hair out prematurely and irritating the skin.

- Conditioners can help to lubricate hair strands after natural oils are removed by shampoos.

- Anti-dandruff shampoos need to be used two to three times per week to keep *Malassezia* yeast at bay.

- Try to limit repeated heat damage to hair by using a diffuser attachment on your hairdryer.

- To increase volume of fine/spare hair apply a mousse to wet hair before drying

- Wait until your hair is completely dry before using flat/curling irons, try to choose irons with ceramic plates and variable temperature settings.

- To protect dry hair before straightening apply a specially formulated heat-resistant protective cream/serum/balm

- For a sleek look after drying/styling apply a high gloss spray. To keep curls longer style your hair (after towel drying) using curlers/Velcro rollers/rags and allow to dry naturally

- Try to ensure your hair is in good condition before colour-treating it.

- If you repeatedly use permanent dark coloured hair dye get a 'skin test' to check you haven't developed an allergy to PPD.

- Have your hair permed/straightened/relaxed at a professional salon if at all possible to get the best outcome for your hair.

CHAPTER 9

Hair Removal, How can we Get Rid of Unwanted Hair?

Does shaving/plucking make our hair grow back stronger and thicker? What are in-growing hairs? Hair removal, what works best, and do home-use hair removal devices actually work? Is laser hair removal effective and safe?

Hair removal is a surprisingly controversial topic. Why should hair be removed at all, when it is naturally occurring on our bodies? Why have different cultures evolved preferences for hair on some areas of the body and not on others? The pressure to remove hair or leave hair to grow has been around for centuries. Enforced hair removal has been used in the past as a way of demeaning slaves, convicts and prisoners of war. In modern military establishments army recruits often have their heads shaved or hair cut very short when they first arrive. Evidently a shaved head acts to remove their individual identity and helps them instead associate with the group and a new way of life. However, voluntary hair removal is a fashion or fad that is continuously changing and evolving in different cultures, social groups and parts of the world.

The subject of beards is an interesting one. Currently they are very fashionable and there has been a recent surge in men growing a beard in Europe and the USA. There is a lot of speculation as to the reasons for this including: fashion statement; looking more 'manly'; shaving is time-consuming; it's an easy way to dramatically change one's appearance. A survey recently conducted by aftershave manufacturers 'Lynx' found that 63% of men thought that beards made a man look more attractive and 'manly' whilst 92% of women questioned said they preferred men without a beard or stubble.

Whatever the fashion is or your opinion, to shave or not to shave is usually a conscious decision for men and women. Shaving daily can be very time consuming and may lead to skin irritation. Men may grow a beard to show their religious beliefs or for convenience or personal preference. Equally they may be required to shave 'clean' for their place of work. The US military for example prohibited any facial hair during the Second World War to try to ensure gas-masks fitted properly.

Whether we like it or not, our outward appearance does say something about us, and beards are no exception. In ancient times, wise men often had long beards which were thought of as a sign of wisdom and virility. In ancient Egypt, many people had all their bodily hair shaved off whilst in contrast, the Pharaohs would usually have a fake beard stuck onto their chins, as a sign of power. By contrast, an unruly beard along with torn clothing and a poor physical state can indicate someone who is from an underprivileged background or may be homeless. A carefully manicured beard/moustache on the other hand can indicate attention to detail and time to spend attaining a particular look.

Hair removal by shaving has been recorded as early as 300BC. Flints, stones, shells and other sharpened materials were used initially, before the advent of bronze, copper and iron. Unearthed tombs in Egypt dating from the 4th millennium BC contained solid gold and copper razors. Frequent shaving however didn't become popular until the 18th century when the wealthy could visit barbershops and let someone else do the work. However, it was not until the advent of disposable safety razors that shaving became mainstream, as it is now, inexpensive, safe and easy to use.

A Mintel survey conducted in the UK in 2014 found that 73% of women and 58% of men said they felt under pressure to remove hair from their bodies. Presumably this pressure is partly cultural and revolves around what is considered to be normal. 8% of women and 30% of men hadn't removed any body hair in the last 12 months. Of the 92% of women undertaking hair removal the most common sites were legs, underarms, pubic region, arms and feet. For men, the most common site for hair removal was the face, followed by the public region, underarms, trunk and buttocks. The frequency of shaving will depend on the desired appearance, but most people shave areas of their face every few days or so.

Have you ever thought that shaving your hair seems to make it grow back thicker and stronger? Then you're not alone, this is a commonly held belief. Numerous studies over the years however have investigated this hypothesis carefully and found that the rate of hair growth and hair diameter is unaltered by shaving. In one of the studies volunteers were asked to shave one of their legs weekly for several months and leave the other. The conclusion was that the act of shaving did not alter the hair growth pattern (hair width, coarseness, rate of growth).

Another myth to the converse is that shaving eyebrow hair stops them growing back. However, a study conducted in 1999, asked volunteers to shave one eyebrow and leave the other. Six months later an independent observer was asked to identify which eyebrow had been shaved, and they found there was no discernible difference between the two brows. You can however stop eyebrow hairs growing back eventually by constantly plucking/threading/waxing a few hairs repeatedly (more of that later).

However, you can see how these myths might arise. For example, when a young man starts shaving his beard area, he will probably recall his hair being fine and downy to start with and over the years it became thicker and coarser. But it's not the shaving that brings about this change, it's the natural hair maturation process, as the fine vellus hairs of childhood are replaced by full thickness terminal hairs. If it was indeed true that shaving our hair made it grow back thicker and stronger, then we would need to increase the frequency of shaving over time, but as we know the frequency stays the same over many years.

Hairs tend to clump together in naturally occurring groups called 'follicular units', where there are between one and four hairs sharing one sebaceous gland and sensory nerves etc. On close inspection after shaving it can appear as if several hairs are coming out of a single follicular opening, leading to the myth that hair density might be increasing, however, these clumps are naturally occurring, in fact, the natural appearance of these follicular units is utilised in hair transplant surgery when the units are transplanted as miniature hair grafts to ensure the hair looks natural afterwards.

If we think of an uncut hair strand being like the branch on a tree; if we cut off the tapered flexible end of the branch then we are left with a short stubby blunt tip that will feel coarse compared to the tapered end we just cut off. When hair starts to grow back after shaving we notice 'stubble' which comprises short hairs sticking straight out of the skin, which can feel quite coarse to the touch.

So shaving our hair doesn't actually affect its growth rate. But what about other hair removal modalities? Interestingly, the answer to this question is that some physical hair removal methods do affect the way the hair may/may not grow back. Plucking hairs, threading, electrolysis, waxing, intense pulsed light and laser hair removal can all lead to some permanent loss of hairs. These methods all affect the hair root, which if damaged may mean the hair can't recover. In some instances, this permanent hair removal is considered to be a bonus.

Recently an intriguing study was published in which scientists showed that if hairs are carefully plucked from the backs of mice, then depending on the density of the plucking, more could grow back than were originally there. They described something called a 'sense and response' phenomenon whereby if sufficient hairs are plucked (above a certain threshold) then this triggered quorum sensing whereby signals were sent out to stimulate increased hair growth. This is a fascinating phenomenon which may or may not have any relevance to human hairs, but nonetheless may point the way to understanding the mechanisms by which we could stimulate hair growth in the future.

There is a condition in humans (often children) where there is a compulsory urge to pull out our hair (usually on the scalp), called trichotillomania. In this condition, usually the same patch of hair is pulled and this leads to progressive hair loss (alopecia) at that site rather than increased hair density. Research shows that the physical pulling of the hair leads to 'split ends' (trichoptilosis), irregular coiled hair and bleeding into the hair follicles. This ultimately damages the hair roots, destroying the hairs' ability to recover. Treatment can involve 'habit reversal' by either face-to-face sessions or self-help via the internet (StopPulling.com).

Many women (including myself) will use plucking or threading to shape their eyebrows. This 'eyebrow epilation' usually involves the use of tweezers or cotton thread looped around the hairs, which are then pulled out. Hairs are pulled out by the root in plucking/threading/waxing and it usually takes four to six weeks for the hair to grow again, which is what makes this method attractive in comparison to shaving. Waxing is usually used in preference to plucking/threading when large areas of hair removal are needed. Some people have observed that repeated physical hair removal over the years eventually leads to less of the hairs growing back and some of the hairs becoming finer downy hairs.

Any physical tugging-out of hairs may cause inflammation around the hair roots (the infundibulum to be precise), which can lead to irreversible damage and permanent hair loss. This physical removal may also lead to folliculitis (redness/bumps around where the hairs come out of the skin), bruising and in-growing hairs.

Pseudofolliculitis (in-grown hair) can lead to pain and disfigurement. There appears to be a genetic predisposition to in-grown hair, with risk factors including men of sub-Saharan African lineage, curly hair, a single-gene substitution in keratin and grooming practices. This is a difficult condition to manage, but a combination of leaving the hair to grow for a while, soothing medicated lotions and ultimately laser hair removal may help.

If physical removal of hair is leading to irritation and folliculitis then chemical depilation could be used instead, so how does this work? Chemical hair removal creams (gels, lotions, aerosols, roll-ons) remove the hair to just beneath the surface of the skin. That is why it takes about a week before the hair is obvious again, unlike shaving when it only takes one or two days. The hair removal creams usually contain calcium or potassium thioglycolate which breaks down the disulphide bonds in the keratin. If left in contact with the hair long enough then eventually this weakens the hair sufficiently, so that it can be 'wiped off' with a cloth.

The strong unpleasant odour of the preparations is due to sulphur-like chemicals that are formed with the thioglycolate reacts with the sodium hydroxide. A similar chemical, ammonium thioglycolate, is used in perms, so it's easy to see if that is left on too long that hair breakage and alopecia could result. These chemical hair removal products are usually cheap, easy to use and are very unlikely to cause skin irritation if used as directed (a small test patch area should be done, before large areas to check for sensitivity), so are an attractive alternative method of hair removal.

More permanent hair removal for some people, is the ultimate goal. Electrolysis has been around for years (first reported use in 1875) and is one of the methods of epilation that can in some cases lead (after multiple treatments) to permanent hair removal. It involves sticking an electrical probe (wire) down into the hair follicle and delivering a shot of electrical current to the hair root. The loosened hair is then removed with tweezers. The risk of infection has been greatly reduced by the introduction of single-use pre-sterilised probes. Hairs in the growing anergen phase of the hair cycle are most likely to be permanently removed; however, not all the hairs will be in anergen at any one time, and therefore some hairs grow back. This is why it is often recommended that hairs are shaved one to five days prior to electrolysis, so that only growing hairs are then targeted. If permanent hair removal is the aim, then 15-30 treatments of electrolysis, usually spaced one to two weeks apart, are required.

The advantages of electrolysis are that it is widely available, it is suitable for all hair colours/types, it is generally pain free (slight tingling only) and it is usually very effective. The disadvantages are costs involved, potential for skin discolouration and possible scarring (if not performed properly) and usually only small areas can easily be tackled. More recently available are home use tweezer epilators which deliver an electric current to the hair near the skin surface. There is currently no significant body of evidence to show these are as effective as traditional electrolysis probes which target hair under the skin surface, but I guess the advantage is that they are cheaper and can be used at home.

Laser hair removal and intense pulsed light (IPL) are more recent additions to the armoury of options available for permanent hair removal. Just like electrolysis, these methods need to be repeated and therefore a course of treatment can be expensive. Large areas can be treated relatively quickly and are thought to be less likely to cause scarring then electrolysis. Lasers usually target the dark brown/black pigment in the hair, therefore they may be less effective in people with very fair hair and those with dark hair and dark skin.

Laser technology is constantly evolving to increase efficacy and reduce potential adverse effects. Alexandrite (755nm), ruby laser (694nm), ND-YAG (1064nm) and diode (800nm) lasers for hair removal have been used successfully for many years. They all work by causing heat damage to the hair follicle by targeting the melanin pigment within it, a process called selective photothermolysis. Longer wavelength lasers have less effect at the skin surface and are therefore thought of as causing less damage to skin pigment.

Permanent hair removal (complete destruction of follicles) is achieved in about 15% to 30% of treated hairs at each treatment. What is commonly seen is temporary hair loss in the treated area as the laser has induced a telogen-like state, which causes the hair to 'rest' before later re-growing. Multiple treatments are therefore required whichever system is used (usually monthly treatments for six months) and at six months 30-50% permanent hair removal is reported. Diode type lasers with low fluence (energy), high power and multiple passes have been found to be slightly superior in some studies to the high energy single pass lasers for long-term hair removal effects.

Potential adverse effects of laser hair removal include discomfort during the treatment, skin redness afterwards, skin pigment change, inflammation and scarring of the skin. All these effects can usually be reduced if a highly-trained individual is carrying out the procedures and they select the appropriate individuals for the appropriate treatment. Those with darker skin tones are at slightly higher risk of developing pigmentary skin changes after treatment.

Home-use laser devices with low fluence are now available to buy for laser hair removal. A study conducted recently in Denmark analysed the efficacy of one such device (810nm laser used at 5.0-6.4 Jcm2) on the growth of axillary hair in women. 36 women of different hair colours were recruited and randomised to either zero or one self-administered treatment each week for eight weeks. Follow-up period extended to three months beyond the last treatment. They showed that during continued treatment reduction in hair growth was 59%, and remaining hairs were 1/3 thinner and 5% lighter in colour. Interestingly on stopping the treatment hair returned to baseline levels within three months and in some cases regrowth exceeded pre-treatment levels, 29% more hair and 7% thicker.

Intense pulsed light (IPL) has become an appealing alternative to lasers for permanent hair removal as it is frequently cheaper and faster. Unlike lasers, which produce a monochromatic single high power (coherent) beam, IPL uses a xenon polychromatic flash lamp with a non-coherent light beam in the visible to infrared light spectrum (ranging from 500–1,200 nm). Because of its wide range of wavelengths IPL can hit multiple targets in the skin, and therefore have potentially multiple uses, but also potentially multiple adverse effects if used by an inexperienced practitioner. Generally speaking, IPL is not advised for those with darker skin tones or those who are tanned as they are more likely to suffer from post-treatment skin pigment changes.

Most studies comparing IPL and laser hair removal show similar efficacy. A recent split-leg study comparing the low fluence multiple pass diode laser (on one leg) and high fluence IPL (on the other leg). Participants had three treatments six to eight weeks apart. At 12 months' results were similar for both treatments, a 75% reduction in hair on both legs with slightly higher pain reported during the IPL treatment.

So what about home-use IPL devices? Home treatment is appealing as it is generally cheaper and more convenient than attending a commercial unit. These home-use devices tend to use a lower fluence than professional machines due to regulatory body concerns about inexperienced operators using them without any specialist guidance. The FDA has currently approved the IPL (475-1,200nm) Silk'n device (Home Skinovations, Kfar Saba, Israel) for home hair removal.

There have been concerns about the need for eye protection and the possibility of skin burns if the devices are used inappropriately but so far these incidents are uncommon. The efficacy of IPL is highly variable between different studies even those using the same device. This may in part be explained by the wide range of wavelengths delivered in a single treatment. Efficacy ranges from 36-64% permanent hair removal at six months' follow-up. So generally, quite promising results.

Top Tips for Hair Removal

- When selecting a hair removal method consider cost, time and desired outcome.

- New electric razors are less likely to cause 'razor rash' and are fast and convenient to use.

- If you develop 'razor bumps' (folliculitis) then consider switching to a less 'close-shave' razor.

- Apply a soothing gel/light cream after shaving to reduce inflammation and irritation.

- Chemical hair removal is a useful alternative to physical hair removal methods if folliculitis is a problem.

- Consider undertaking a 'test patch' area before removing hair over a large expanse of skin.

- Shave your hair one to five days prior to electrolysis so that only active growing hairs are treated.

- Always check the qualifications and experience of anyone offering laser/IPL hair removal.

Tips to reduce skin irritation from shaving

- Wet shaving causes less irritation than electric/dry shaving

- Use warm water rather than cold

Use a shaving gel and make a rich thick lather over the area to be shaved

- Use a razor with 3 blades

The first pass of the razor should be 'with the hair' (rather than against them)

After first shaving in the direction of hair growth then reapply more gel and shave against the direction of growth (second pass)

- Apply a soothing 'after-shave' gel or lotion

If you are prone to shaving rashes, then use this way of shaving alternate days

CHAPTER 10

Nails

What helps them grow strong? How can our nails reflect underlying illnesses? Does manicuring nails damage them? Why do our nails change at different stages of our lives? How can we improve the strength of our nails?

Many years ago physicians used to just study the hands of their patients and from that they were able to diagnose numerous underlying conditions. This skill seemed to have an almost magical quality about it, which allowed the physician to just look at the hands and from that see into the patient's very soul. Even today you can tell a lot by looking at someone's hands, and particularly their nails, which may give an indication of underlying internal illnesses. Modern medical doctors will still often start their examinations by looking at the nails, because their appearance is a rich source of medical information. But to be able to recognise when something is wrong, we first need to know what 'normal' is, and that can be different at different ages. So if you will bear with me, a little anatomy and biochemistry first.

Finger and toe nails are made of hard keratin, similar to the material used to make claws/horns and hooves in animals. Apart from regular cutting of our nails and occasional decoration, most of us pay little attention to them, unless they start malfunctioning. Nails are designed to protect the ends of our fingers and toes from micro trauma associated with walking/running and handling numerous objects on an everyday basis. Finger nails also help us to pick up very fine objects. But how much do we know about our nails, how they grow and why/how they can become diseased?

To understand nail growth, we need to know a little about nail structure.

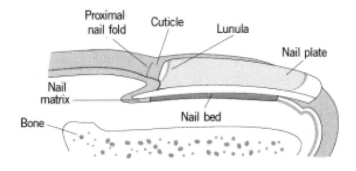

The nail plate is the hard bit of the nail that is connected to the skin by the cuticle which is cemented down to the nail matrix. 25% of the nail plate is actually found underneath the proximal nail fold – so this helps to anchor the nail. We can usually see the pink colour of our nail bed through the nail plate as the bed has a rich blood-vessel supply. The cuticle is actually attached to the proximal nail fold skin and is there to act as a seal or barrier to germs getting in under the skin. Pushing back the cuticle too much as part of manicuring can damage the cuticle, leading to inflammation and infection.

Fingernails grow about twice as quickly as toenails, and the longer the finger (or toe) the more rapid the growth of the nail. So our middle fingernail grows faster than our thumb/little finger nails. The average rate of growth of most fingernails is 4.8mm/month and toenails 2mm/month. If you have ever damaged your nail plate such as hitting it with a hammer, you will notice it take months for the blood patch in the nail to 'grow-out'. On average it take nine months to grow a new finger nail and 12-14 months to grow a new toenail.

If we are seriously ill for a few weeks or more, our nails can temporarily stop growing and then when we recover they start growing again. The episode of nail growth arrest is subsequently seen in all our nails as a horizontal line called Beau's line which corresponds to when we were ill. A bit like rings on a tree trunk showing good or bad growing seasons, whereas unlike tree rings the Beau's line will eventually grow out.

As we get older the thickness of our nail plate increases. You may have noticed that babies have quite soft thin nails that can look a bit curved, medics call then 'spoon' nails (Koilonychia) as they are convex in the middle. You might also have noticed that you have to cut babies' nails regularly as they seem to grow very rapidly. Older people by contrast have much thicker nails that may be difficult to cut. You may also start to notice longitudinal ridges (onychorrhexis, senile nails) especially on your thumb nails once you get past the age of 50 years. These ridges can also be seen in rheumatoid arthritis and iron deficiency anaemia.

Factors affecting nail plate growth according to Mefford and colleagues include; nutritional status, environmental temperature (faster growth in the warmth), trauma, pregnancy, acute illness, skin disease and handedness (faster growth of the nails on the dominant side). I can't say I have ever noticed my nails growing faster in the summer months, but I expect I don't pay much attention to them.

So what nutritional factors affect nail growth? There are lots of products in the chemist and the supermarket claiming to help growth healthy nails, but what is the evidence? Probably not very much is the short answer. Double blind placebo controlled trials of nail products are few and far between. To date there is nothing available that seems to increase the rate of nail growth: however, some preparations do claim to reduce the fragility of our nails. Once the nail plate emerges from the cuticle, it is dead tissue so it would be very difficult to influence that in terms of growth by applying preparations to the nail plate itself. However, reducing its dryness and flakiness could be possible by using rich emollient products, in a similar way to hair products applied to dry and damaged hair.

Nails (and hair) are made from a protein called keratin and the hardness of the nail plate is related to the concentration of sulphur matrix proteins. 90% of the nail consists of 'hard keratin' and 10% 'soft keratin'. The overall sulphur content is about 10%, which helps to form the strong disulphide bonds which basically glue the keratin fibres together.

Because keratin is so important to the strength of hair and nails, some researchers in the USA/Australia decided to make a super-concentrated oral supplement of keratin and test it to see if it helped fragile/broken hair and nails. The product Cynatine HNS was provided by the manufacturing company Roxlor Global (the lead researcher in the study, RH Veghte, was also the general manager of this company), so we need to bear this in mind when we look at the results, as there is the potential for bias interpretation. Having said that, the study, which was conducted in 2014, was a randomised, double-blinded placebo controlled trial.

They recruited 50 women between the ages of 40-71 years with 'stressed/damaged hair' and their nails were also assessed by the researchers. They gave half of the women placebo capsules and half Cynatine capsules for 90 days. Most of the results relate to improvement in hair strength/reduced hair loss. However,

they also assessed the participants' nails for breakage, fragility and smoothness/colour. They did find that compared to the placebo group 87% of the women taking the keratin capsules had 'hard nails' by day 90 with a significant reduction in nail breakage compared to the placebo group. There was also significant improvement in the smoothness and white colour of the nails.

So, it does look as if oral supplements of keratin can help nail hardness, bearing in mind the small number of women in the study and the manufacturer's involvement in the research.

But what about calcium supplements which are often included in nail products, is there any evidence that they help? It seems quite logical to imagine that calcium would make our nails stronger as we know that nails do contain some calcium, and that calcium makes bones stronger, but can we really make that link? The amount of calcium in nails is actually only 0.3% which is a tiny proportion of its total composition when you compare it to bones, which contain 20-25% calcium. So adding calcium to our diet may make our bones stronger, but what about nails? Well, contrary to popular belief there is little evidence that calcium contributes to nail hardness. Levels of calcium do tend to be slightly higher in older people compared to children, and they are generally higher in men.

Few actual studies exist formally looking at calcium and nails. However, one study conducted at Auckland University in 2000, examined 683 healthy postmenopausal women taking part in a randomized placebo-controlled trial of calcium supplements (1g Calcium citrate per day) for the prevention of osteoporosis. The women were around the age of 70 years and had normal dietary calcium intake of around 800-1200mg per day. The women took the additional calcium supplements for one year. At the end of the study the women were then asked to score the changes in their finger and toe nails – including brittleness and texture. Women in the placebo and the calcium groups noted no change in their nails during the study period. So, no evidence here from self-reported nail quality that calcium improves the appearance of our nails.

We also see adverts telling us to take supplements containing iron and zinc to help form strong nails, but are these nutrients actually important for nail growth? Iron is actually needed for strong nails as we know that patients deficient in iron, some of whom may also be anaemic, start to develop spoon shaped, concave nails (Koilonychia). This same clinical sign can be normal in infants under the age of two years, but in older children and adults can indicate low iron levels. However, recent studies have also shown that individuals identified as having iron-deficiency anaemia from a blood test may have normal looking nails which contain normal levels of iron. So some people seem to be able to maintain the iron level in their nails, even though their serum iron levels are low.

Similarly, patients with zinc deficiency in their blood had normal zinc levels in their nails. So somehow the body is able to maintain normal levels of these nutrients in the nails despite deficiency elsewhere in the body. So most of us won't know if our nails are deficient or not as there is no routine test available.

So does what we take in orally actually affect our nail plate composition? Well, a recent paediatric dental study in Brazil examining the composition of their finger and toenails found that the amount of fluoride used in the 18-30-month-old infants' toothpastes correlated well with the amount of fluoride in their nails. So, another benefit from brushing twice daily with a fluoride containing toothpaste could be stronger nails in children.

So overall there is little evidence that taking supplements has much effect on the texture and strength of our nails. But, what about products that are designed to be rubbed onto the nail plates directly and the surrounding skin? Well, there is some evidence that rubbing lipid rich moisturisers onto dry nails can enhance their hydration and reduce brittleness. Lipids made up of glycolic and stearic acids help to keep nails water resistant, keeping water levels of nails around 18%. If the water content of our nails drops below 16% nails can become brittle and above 25% they become soft.

So if it's not calcium contributing to nail hardness what other minerals might be important? Well there is evidence that magnesium and selenium levels do affect the likelihood of nail splitting and flaking. However, the actual mineral content of the nails is different between males and females and the young and the old. Generally, neonates have the highest levels of iron in their nails, then children, and lowest of all levels occurs in adult nails. Children also tend to have higher levels of magnesium and selenium in their nails. But, as we know children's nails are usually softer than adult nails, so minerals are important but they are less likely to contribute to nail strength than keratins and sulphur.

Most of us will never have our nails analysed for deficiencies so what we need to rely on more is the appearance of our nails to tell us if all is well. Sometimes we can see discolouration that might cause alarm, but what is normal and what is not?

A common finding when we look at our nails are white spot or streaks. It's a common misconception that this is due to calcium deficiency, but in fact it is cause by micro-trauma to the nail plates, little knocks and bumps, and is completely harmless. If the entire nail plate is white (leukonychia) then this on the other hand may be an indication of an underlying problem with our liver or kidneys, or may relate to medications (such as chemotherapy, steroids and cyclosporine).

Yellow nails usually indicate that the nail plates are very thickened, such as may be seen in older persons, but can also be seen in so-called 'yellow-nail syndrome'. In the latter, there may be underlying lung problems, endocrine disorders and immunodeficiency (when the immune system is lowered for any reason).

Red nails can be observed when there are underlying problems with the heart, rheumatological conditions, kidney and liver disorders. We often also see red streaks in the nails – particularly at the free edge and these are called splinter haemorrhages, they are more common in people who undertake manual work (from micro trauma) but may also indicate an underlying infective endocarditis (infection of the heart valves).

Blue nails may be associated with medications such as antimalarial, minocycline antibiotic and chemotherapy.

Brown or black discolouration in a nail plate can cause alarm. Trauma to the nail can result in bleeding under the nail, which initially can look red or purple, then black and finally brown, and this discolouration will slowly grow out of the nail. If you look closely you will see that there is a sort of bruise under the nail and sometimes a horizontal white line next to it depicting the traumatic event. Bleeding under the nail is not normally a problem; however, if it is very acute and there is a large volume then it can be very painful and very occasionally this needs to be released surgically by boring a hole through the nail plate to let the blood out.

Melanonychia or brown colour is usually due to an actual pigment in the nail rather than a result of blood, and may be associated with a naevus (mole) causing pigment in the nail matrix, or may suggest a fungal infection of the nail. Those with dark skin can commonly have pigmented lines in their nails (linear melanonychia), which are harmless. What is more worrying, however, is when the pigment under the nail becomes wider, more irregular and spills onto the skin around the nail (Hutchinson's sign) which can indicate a melanoma (cancerous mole) under the nail.

This type of melanoma is not thought to be related to sun exposure, but is more likely to be related to trauma and is most common on the big toe or thumb. Because this type of skin cancer is usually under the toenail – a place we rarely look - it often presents late when the tumour may have already spread into the blood/lymphatics. The famous reggae singer Bob Marley reportedly injured his right big toe whilst playing soccer, the injury did not heal properly and eventually he was diagnosed with melanoma of the same toenail. Some experts think the trauma was not the cause and that the melanoma was already present, but it is always difficult to know. Doctors advised Marley to have an amputation, which on religious grounds he declined and eventually the cancer spread to his brain and internal organs. He tragically died four years later, aged 36 years.

Melanoma under the nail often presents late to the doctor as it is frequently not seen or recognised as a potential problem by healthcare professionals. Some of the melanomas are not even pigmented which can make the diagnosis even more difficult to make for GPs and dermatologists alike.

If the nail plate starts to become 'un-glued' from the nail bed then it can start lifting up which can be a real nuisance. The loose edge starts to snag on clothing and it can be painful if yanked accidentally. The lifting up of the nail gives it a kind of 'oil drop' appearance. The nail plate is no longer translucent where it is lifting up and looks more opaque and can be slightly yellowish or salmon coloured. This can be a sign of micro-trauma of the toenails – often seen in keen runners and footballers- or may indicate psoriasis or fungal infection of the nails.

The extreme form of this phenomenon, is complete shedding of the nails called onychomadesis. This can be caused by major trauma but also may result from underlying arsenic or lead poisoning.

One of the oldest clinical signs of the nails was documented by Hippocrates in the 5th century BC where he described increased longitudinal curvature of the nail called 'clubbing' (nothing to do with going out on a Saturday night!). Clubbing can be inherited: however, if acquired in later life can indicate serious underlying disease. This is a classic medical student question in exams – 'list five causes of clubbing', (lung disease such as chronic obstructive pulmonary disease, lung cancer; heart conditions such as bacterial endocarditis and congenital heart disease; gut problems like ulcerative colitis/Crohn's disease and liver cirrhosis, thyroid conditions and even pregnancy).

Brittle nails are a common complaint and this can be associated with rough sand-paper like nail plates, fragile split ends and ridges. This trachyonychia has been associated with biotin deficiency (which can occur due to an imbalance of gut bacteria and taking antibiotics/anti-epileptic medicines). Biotin supplements of 2.5mg daily for six to 12 months in a study did result in a 25% increased thickness of the nail plates of those with brittle nails. Biotin also known as vitamin H or vitamin B_7 is produced in large amounts by gut bacteria so deficiency of biotin is very rare. Biotin is also found in peanuts, leafy green vegetables and liver. Supplements are rarely needed; however, biotin is often added to hair/nail products due to some evidence that it can cause strengthening.

Cutting our nails seems to be straightforward enough. Get a pair of nail scissors or clippers and trim away the free edge of the nail plate to the desired level. However, it can be a difficult process for some. Have you ever tried to cut a baby's nails? Tricky when they are squirming about. In fact, my husband (also a doctor) managed to cut our second son's toe in the delivery suite, attempting to cut his nails, aged one hour! (sorry Blake!) There was a lot of screaming from Blake and the midwife at my husband. Older people who have very thick nail plates can also struggle to cut their nails, particularly if they are not as flexible and dextrous as they once were in terms of reaching down to their toes and scissors may not be strong enough to cut through the thick keratin.

Quite a common problem is so called 'in-growing' toenails. This usually affects the great toes, and frequently starts after the nails have been cut too short, or in those of us who have a tendency to develop pincer shaped nails. As the nails grow back following trimming, the nail plate grows into the fleshy skin at the sides of the nail. This causes a lot of pain and inflammation, and some people find it hard to wear shoes or even walk because of the pain. I have seen one patient who also had in-growing fingernails from cutting the nails too aggressively down the sides of the nail plates. Management of in-growing nails can be conservative or surgical. I mention the conservative ones here, as you can do these yourself at home, and they can be very effective.

There are various conservative methods used to try to help 'in-growing' toenails, including application of antiseptics such as hydrogen peroxide and potassium permanganate to the inflamed skin. Phenol may be applied to the affected area to 'toughen up' the vulnerable skin. Toe braces have recently come back into fashion and in studies have been shown to get people back to work faster than those who opt for surgical removal of their toenails. The toenail brace is fitted and bonded horizontally across the distal part of the affected nail plate, which helps to reduce the curvature of the nail and therefore relieve the pressure on the skin.

Recent studies have also shown that taping the skin down along the sides of the nail can also help the recovery process and reduce pain. Here's how to do it: -

Take a piece of adhesive flexible tape/Elastoplast (about 3cm by 2.5cm) and run it parallel to the affected side/s of the toenail. As you apply the tape to the skin at the sides of the nail, put it under tension and pull the fold of skin outwards away from the nail. If you look on-line you can see diagrams and video's showing you how to do this in detail. Taping needs to be done daily for it to work. Because toenails grow relatively slowly, this taping will need to be carried out daily for six to eight weeks. So a slow and laborious process but hugely preferable for many of those affected, than needing to having the toenails removed surgically or to suffer ongoing pain. Once the nail has grown back over the skin, rather than digging into it, ensure only conservative nail trimming in the future to try to prevent recurrence.

Apart from cutting our toenails, some of us like to have manicures or pedicures. But do these help our nails in terms of function or are they basically cosmetic? There is no doubt that keeping our nails finely trimmed means they are less likely to snag and fracture due to micro-trauma of daily activities. And it can be very relaxing and helpful to have an expert cut and polish your nails. Nail strengthening polishes and hydrating our nails can help to protect them from friction. Podiatrists and chiropodists are trained in the art of toenail cutting, which may not be offered as part of a finger/toe nail manicure.

Over-manicuring our nails on the other hand can be associated with nail and skin damage. Instrumentation can cause abrasion, nail polish remover and nail polish itself can leave nails feeling rough, brittle and even thinned. A report three years ago from Florida described five women who developed severe thinning of their nails after using a new manicure system that involved the use of gel polish and removal with acetone and manual peeling. They all developed white steaks on their nails from the minor trauma.

Nail bars are springing up everywhere with 'nail art' becoming one of the fastest growth industries in the cosmetic arena in the last few years. Artificial (acrylic) nails can be 'glued' on to our nail plates for a perfectly manicured nail appearance with no cracking or splitting. However there have been reports of fungal infections getting under the false nails. Allergic contact dermatitis to acrylates used to be seen only in dentists, printers and fibreglass workers: however, currently nail technicians are the occupational group most commonly affected. There are even recent reports of nail glue adhesive, which can get up to temperatures of 68°C, causing full thickness skin burns. So make sure you go to a nail bar with a good reputation.

And finally, a word about fish pedicures. They seem to be all the rage, particularly in holiday resorts. If you can get over the fear/excitement of putting your feet in a bowl of fish-filled water, then the little team of cleaners nibble away at dead skin cells and give your feet a really good clean. What could go wrong? Well, most of the time, not a lot! But there have been reports of skin infections resulting from fish pedicures when the fish have been carrying bacteria such as *Staphylococcus aureus*, even MRSA (the resistant form) and a mycobacterial infection that some fish might be carrying. So check the fish look healthy before taking the plunge.

Top Nail Tips

• Ensure you cut your nails carefully and don't trim them too short. Little and often is best.

• If you are struggling to cut your own toenails, ask for help from relatives or healthcare professionals such as podiatrists and chiropodists.

- Don't push back your cuticles too much as this can damage them and let in infection.

- If you eat a healthy diet and are generally fit, it is unlikely that you need to take hair/nail supplements.

- If your nails are brittle and rough, rub hydrating cream into your nails, eat more leafy greens and peanuts or consider taking biotin.

- If you see colour changes in your nails or changes in nail curvature, ask your doctor to take a look.

- Gentle polishing and buffing of the nails can help to keep them smooth, but over-manicuring should be avoided.

- Nail art can look amazing, but be aware of allergies and infections that might occur.

CHAPTER 11

Scars and Wound Healing

How does the skin heal itself? What are the risk factors for poor skin healing? Do different skin sites have different healing properties? Why do I develop bumpy scars? What can I do to minimise the appearance of a scar after an injury/operation?

The skin is the largest organ in the body, whose main function is to protect our delicate insides, so when it's under attack it needs to respond rapidly to repair any damage. Trauma, burns and surgery all damage the skin, setting off an automatic chain reaction of spontaneous healing. This healing process is a complex series of events and both under-healing and over-healing can lead to problems, so the balance is critical to minimising the resultant scar.

If only the very top layer of the skin (epidermis) is affected by trauma, then there is no bleeding and the skin heals very rapidly with no residual marks. However, if the deeper layer of the skin (dermis) is damaged then there will be bleeding and ultimately a scar may form. It is estimated that 100 million people in the developed world acquire scars following surgery each year, and of those 15% will develop an 'overgrown' or unsightly scar.

Scars can cause physical and psychological problems. You may have experienced the itching and tenderness of a fresh scar and ultimately some of us will develop a stiff and even contracted scar. Psychological effects of scars that are perceived as unsightly include anxiety, low self-esteem and even depression. So trying to ensure that skin heals in the best possible way after trauma, surgery and burns can make a huge difference to the outcome.

There are three main stages of skin healing: an inflammatory phase (where the body immediately responds to the assault); the proliferative phase (when the skin is rebuilt) and finally a maturation phase (which can continue for up to two years after the skin has closed over).

When the skin is traumatized the inflammatory phase of wound healing is triggered. Cells called platelets (which are sticky cells in the blood stream) clump together to plug the hole and stop the bleeding. Proteins in the blood (fibrin and plasma) join the platelets to shore up the breach and they help to form a scab. At the same time the blood vessels in the area dilate to allow white cells, growth factors and other nutrients to come into the skin. At this stage the wound often looks red and swollen. The proliferation phase starts when skin fibroblast cells are activated in the wound and they start producing collagen (fibrous tissue), which along with a cement type of material (extra-cellular matrix) rebuild the damaged skin.

New skin cells start forming from the bottom of a superficial wound and from the edge of a deep wound and slowly they start closing the gap until the new skin has completely formed. Once the wound looks completely healed up from the outside then the two-year maturation process starts, which slowly over time remodels the tissue underneath the skin surface.

Generally, as scars mature they become paler and flatter: however, sometimes scars can become stretched, depressed, bumpy (hypertrophic) or even form large lumps way beyond the original injury (keloid scar). Keloid scars feel very firm because they are made up of dense fibrous collagen. What makes the fibroblasts keep on producing collagen long after the wound has healed over, is poorly understood: however, there is evidence it's to do with over production and increased activity of growth factors.

Certain areas of the body appear to be high risk sites for hypertrophic/keloid scars, such as the front of the chest, the back of the shoulders and the earlobes. It does seem strange that some areas of the body are more susceptible to poor healing than others, but continuous stretching tension on the skin is thought to be a factor in triggering keloids.

There also appears to be a genetic predisposition to forming large scars. Black and Asian skin types seem to have a much higher rate of keloid formation than Caucasian or Mediterranean skin types. Women are more commonly affected than men and older people are more at risk than younger. One research paper published in the USA 10 years ago showed that keloid formation on the earlobe after ear-piercing was more likely to occur if the person was over the age of 11 years and if there was a family history of keloids.

The lower legs are often also a site of poor healing as the blood supply is quite sluggish and the skin tends to be thin and under pressure when standing. Healing can be very slow, particularly in older people with papery-thin skin. This is often why lower leg ulcers take many weeks or months to heal up.

Scar prevention manoeuvres can start well in advance of planned surgery: however, many of us will sustain unexpected trauma or burns where pre-planning is not possible. It's generally been shown that to minimise the appearance of scars we should try to reduce tension on the wound edges. Surgeons try to achieve this by making their skin incisions parallel to skin tension lines. Any crust or crud that sticks to the top of the wound should be gently removed by washing with a mild disinfectant.

Contrary to what I was told when I was a kid ('keep it dry'), we now know that keeping the wound surface moist is best for healing. Plain clean Vaseline smeared onto the wound and covered is ideal. Alternatively, silicone dressings and gels can be applied to wounds with good evidence of improved wound comfort and improved healing. Water has been shown to evaporate more rapidly from scars even after one year, compared to the skin around them, so restoring fluid and using an emollient barrier cream can help if used for months afterwards.

Pressure dressings have been shown in studies to help reduce the likelihood of hypertrophic and keloid scars in high risk sites, such as the earlobes and chest. These can be used for up to three months if necessary. Other studies have shown that if silicone dressings are used and additional pressure is applied, then there is even less chance of developing a keloid or hypertrophic scar in those of us at high risk of developing bumpy scars.

If despite this hypertrophic scars still form, then the continued application of silicone dressings is recommended. These are quite expensive, so should be left in place for several days before being washed and reused if possible. If further thickening of the scar continues or a keloid forms then a series of steroid injections can be very helpful, although the injections can be somewhat painful and may bleach the skin slightly.

If keloids don't respond to any of that, then cutting them out under local anaesthetic can be done, but there is a high risk of the keloid recurring afterwards, which is not surprising as they are triggered by skin trauma. After cutting out the keloid, various things have been tried to stop them coming back including pressure dressings, steroid injections, radiotherapy/electron beam and imiquimod cream (which activates interferon leading to a breakdown in collagen). Some of these manoeuvres can help, but recurrence can still occur.

Recently some doctors have tried treating keloids with internal cryotherapy – when a very cold metal rod is inserted into the centre of the keloid and this starts to kill the scar cells from the inside. Early results are promising, with 50% reduction in scar size at 18 months after one treatment.

So what else can you do to help wounds heal better? Stopping smoking around the time of a planned surgical procedure can be extremely helpful. Many dermatology/plastic and maxillofacial surgeons will recommend you stop smoking prior to and after facial surgery to help wounds to heal well.

You may be surprised to hear that tobacco smoke contains about 4000 different compounds including known carcinogens (cancer causing chemicals). I won't list them all here but some of the chemicals in smoke include poisons such as arsenic, carbon monoxide, hydrogen cyanide and polonium. These not only go into your mouth, throat and lungs, they also affect the skin, particularly of the head and neck.

So how do these chemicals affect wound healing? Well, basically they cause lack of oxygen to the tissues, due to shutting down of blood vessels. This affects the ability of cells to function properly and wound healing is consequently impaired. So another good reason to stop smoking! Your doctor can advise you on how to stop smoking and many have smoking cessation support teams who can prescribe nicotine patches or switch to vaping to help you quit.

Other risk factors for poor wound healing include obesity. There are several studies that have shown if you have a high body mass index (BMI) and more fat under your skin you are more likely to have delayed wound healing. Scientists have looked at the reasons for this and have identified that there are less stretchy elastic fibres in the skin above areas where fat cells are enlarged. The elastic fibres are an essential part of wound healing and having less of them around delays wound closure.

Most of us will have some sort of surgical procedure at some point in our lives that will involve cutting through our skin. So you might be surprised to hear that currently there is no consensus amongst surgeons as to whether it is best to keep wounds dry and covered after surgery for a few days/weeks or whether it is best to start washing wounds the next day. There are generally two schools of thought. One is that early washing could help patients to get back to normal more quickly and wash any germs/dirt/sweat off the wounds. And the other is that early washing may lead to poor wound healing, through irritation and maceration (making the skin soggy and fragile).

A Cochrane review (a study which examines all the published studies) conducted in 2015 tried to answer this question about when is the optimum time after an operation to start washing/wetting the wound. It examined hundreds of studies, but only one trial met its strict criteria for consideration. This single trial randomised 857 patients who had a simple excision (something small was cut out of the skin, and the wound was sutured/stitched) in primary care into two groups. One group would wash the wound after 12 hours and the other after 48 hours. The results showed that there was no difference in the infection rates at the surgical site in the two groups, which was overall 8.5% (pretty low). So it's not clear what is best. Most dermatologists opt for early washing of wounds at either 24 or 48 hours and then ask people to apply Vaseline to the fresh wound daily.

But is cheap Vaseline really the best topical preparation to apply to wounds? What about Manuka honey, aloe vera, bio-oil etc.? So what's the evidence? Currently there is a lack of good quality research into the use of these products, making it difficult to answer the question: however, it is fair to say that there is certainly no compelling evidence that aloe vera topical agents or dressings help acute or chronic wound healing (Cochrane review 2012).

Honey has been used for thousands of years as a wound dressing, but it's only recently that its active biological properties have been uncovered. Honey is acidic, and it is this acidity which reduces the activity of proteases which would normally break down proteins. So stopping the breakdown of proteins helps wound healing. Honey also helps to draw fluid out of wounds, which can be helpful if they are very wet and weepy, but less so if they are dry.

Manuka honey (produced in New Zealand) has been much prized and promoted for its ability to kill bacteria which can be helpful in keeping a wound clean and free from infection. But is Manuka honey any better at killing bacteria than just standard honey? Manuka honey can cost from £10-£40, whereas standard honey sells for around £2-£10 per pot. All honey contains hydrogen peroxide (a natural bleach) which kills bacteria, but unfortunately a lot of this activity is neutralised by catalase (an enzyme) which is present in wound tissues. Manuka honey has an additional antibacterial agent called methylglyoxal which is not deactivated by the catalase. So it would seem that Manuka honey probably does have more sustainable antibacterial properties when used on wounds than standard honey.

However, is Manuka honey superior to plain Vaseline? A study conducted in 2006 compared Manuka honey dressings with paraffin (Vaseline) impregnated dressings in 100 patients following toenail surgery. Patients were randomised to receive one of the two dressings, and the time for total healing of the toenail wound was observed. The average healing time if the whole nail was removed was 40.30 days for the honey group and 39.98 days for the paraffin group. So no difference at all. But when they looked at patients who had only had part of their nail removed they healed significantly faster with the paraffin dressing compared to the honey one (19.62 vs 31.76 days). So if anything in this setting, cheap Vaseline was just as good, if not better than the expensive Manuka honey dressing (good news for the cash-strapped NHS).

Many of my patients mention that that have bought 'bio-oil' to apply to any cuts/grazes, stretch marks and surgical wounds. But is there any evidence that it helps in wound healing and minimises the appearance of scars? When you look at the ingredients it basically looks like perfumed mixed oils. The main oils include PurCellin, chamomile, lavender, rosemary and calendula plus vitamins A and E.

The company suggests that the novel PurCellin oil is effective at improving the appearance of scars. But what is PurCellin oil? Well, it's actually a synthetic form of preening oil produced by ducks to keep their feathers water-tight and keep them afloat. When you look at their published study (which only had 37 participants) they claim that after eight weeks 92% showed improvement in the appearance of the scars compared to placebo. But there is no detail as to what the placebo was, what the improvement was and what type of scars were being treated. So, it's difficult to know what to make of these claims, as we know newer scars including stretch marks tend to fade naturally with time. This is an area of research that needs a lot more attention in the future, so we can apply proper 'evidence-based' medicine.

Conventional advice is to ensure you don't get too much sun on new scars. The thinking behind this is that the pale skin in the scar is more vulnerable to sunburn and therefore more at risk for developing a skin cancer.

So usually we recommend that scars are protected with SPF 50 sunscreen for at least one year. There are however some studies that show delivering UVB light to pale/white scars can help them to become darker and therefore less obvious compared to the surrounding skin. So overall, with safety in mind, it is probably best to protect new scars for a year from the sun, but then after that a little bit of sun can help them to darken and blend with your normal skin.

We know that tension on the skin causes stretching of scars, but how does stretching of the skin lead to 'stretch mark' scars? Many of us may have experienced ourselves or know others who have developed stretch marks (striate) at some point in their lives. Striae can form if the skin suddenly gets stretched due to sudden growth. They are not uncommon in teenagers who suddenly put on a 'growth spurt' leading to striae on their back which are perpendicular to the direction of growth. Also, if we put on a lot of weight suddenly for any reason, such as pregnancy, then the skin under the most tension can also develop stretch marks. They usually appear as red streaks to start with and then the colour fades with time to pale.

A study in 2015 took skin biopsies from women with newly formed stretch marks in pregnancy (striae gravidarum, SG) and their normal skin (at the hip). When the two skin samples were compared, they found that in the striae the network of elastic fibres was markedly disrupted compared to the normal skin. Also there were thin, short thread-like structures called fibrils that weren't forming normal elastic fibres. So, what causes some women to develop stretch marks in pregnancy? Identified risk factors in a study conducted in Poland in 2015 showed that your risk of developing them is higher if you have a family history of SG, if you have a high BMI prior to pregnancy, if you have a high birth weight baby and if you have any form of chronic disease. Several studies have also shown that if you do have SG then you are more likely to develop perineal tears during vaginal deliveries than those without stretch marks.

But is there a way of preventing stretch marks in pregnancy developing in the first place? The University of Michigan analysed all the research papers in 2015 and sadly, found that there was no strong reliable evidence from robust studies to show that any topical cream (centella cream [derived from a herbaceous plant], bitter almond oil, olive oil and cocoa butter) can prevent or reduce the severity of SG. There was only some weak evidence to suggest hyaluronic acid may prevent SG.

Another area of our bodies that can have problems with 'wounds' are the insides of our mouths, or aphthous ulcers. Minor abrasions sustained whilst brushing our teeth or eating food can lead to these mouth ulcers forming. They are very common and are small round/oval painful erosions, where the top layer of cells has come off. In the mouth the top layer is very thin, so this kind of erosion occurs relatively easily.

Sometimes however, there is no history of trauma inside the mouth before they appear. People have recognised for many years that they seem to be more common when we are 'run down'. There is certainly evidence that they are also more common when we are stressed, if we have an underlying immune disorders, malabsorption and certain types of vitamin deficiencies. There is thought to be a genetic link leading to this inflammatory reaction in the mucosa. These types of aphthous ulcers seem to be quite common in children and slightly more common in women than men. They tend to occur in groups, a few appearing at a time, and they usually take about a week to heal up.

If you have a tendency to develop mouth ulcers then it may be helpful to use a soft, small headed toothbrush to reduce trauma whilst brushing your teeth. There are lots of products available that can be bought over the counter to try to speed healing of the ulcers. However most of the evidence points towards topical corticosteroids and topical antibiotics being the most effective. In reality most of us will buy a paste or gel to apply to the ulcers to help numb the pain and antiseptic to kill germs that might be getting into the ulcerated area. The gel seems to form a protective barrier over the ulcers and gives some relief, so if they help you to eat, sleep and function whilst they are healing then they are worth using.

Risk Factors for Poor Wound Healing

- Cigarette smoking.
- High BMI.
- Older age.
- Diabetes.
- Poor nutritional state.

Factors helping wound healing and scar appearance

- Wash the new wound daily with a mild antiseptic solution.
- Keep the wound surface moist (paraffin, silicone).
- Use SPF 50 sunscreen to a new scar for one year.
- Avoid stretching the skin at the scar site if possible.
- Use silicone dressings or silicone gel daily to reduce bumpiness.

Risk Factors for Keloid/Hypertrophic Scar Formation

- Those with darker skin tones are more at risk of developing bumpy scars.
- Keloid scars are more common in Africans and Asians than Caucasians.

- High risk skin sites for bumpy scars include the ears, anterior chest, shoulders and upper back.

- Poor healing wounds which may be infected/inflamed.

Risk Factors for Mouth (Aphthous) Ulcers

- Young age, children and adolescents.

- Female.

- Vigorous teeth brushing which causes micro-trauma to gums.

- Poorly fitting dentures/braces.

- Malnutrition, stress, immune disorders.

CHAPTER 12

The Truth about Skin Cancer

What are the real risks factors for developing skin cancer? Is there anything we can do to prevent it? Is it really all down to the sun? What are the signs of skin cancer that we need to look out for? What is the treatment?

Skin cancer is the most common cancer in the world, and accounts for 75% of all cancer diagnoses. Most of us now know that we need to be careful in the sun. However, when I was a child (about 40 years ago) sunburn and the subsequent skin peeling was just part of our normal summer. My brothers and sister and I used to joke amongst ourselves that we were 'ap-pealing' (meaning our skin was peeling post sun exposure)!

Most of us when travelling abroad to sunny climates can immediately sense that the sun is much stronger and we usually take extra care. But what about the sun in the UK and Ireland, is it really as weak as we think or in fact is it intense enough to cause skin cancer? Skin Cancer

Research UK estimate that 86% of skin cancer diagnosed in the UK is linked to UV radiation from the sun. Many of us will have experienced sunburn from sunshine in the UK.

Worldwide there are three main types of skin cancer: Melanoma (malignant melanoma/cancerous moles); Basal cell carcinoma (rodent ulcers, so-called as they slowly 'eat away' the affected skin); and squamous cell carcinoma (a rapidly growing scaly lump).

Melanoma is the most deadly form of skin cancer. Five times as many people in 2015 in the UK had melanoma diagnosed compared to 40 years ago. It's currently the third most common cancer in those aged 15-39 years. In Ireland in both males and females and across all age groups melanoma is the third most common cancer diagnosed.

In the USA in Caucasians the lifetime risk of melanoma is one in 35 men and one in 54 women and in the UK one in 55 for males/females, which is so much lower when compared to Australia where the lifetime risk is one in 14 in males and one in 22 for females. Australia is called the 'sunburn country', as the intensity of the sun is much stronger there than pretty much anywhere else in the world.

Men are more likely to be diagnosed with melanoma than women (67% higher chance) and when diagnosed their prognosis (outlook) is worse with 136% higher risk of dying from melanoma than women. The worse prognosis in men is mainly due to the fact that they present later to their doctor with a problem. Having an abnormal mole on your back often goes unnoticed until someone else points it out, and then it requires making an appointment to see the doctor to get it checked.

Many men in my clinic have been badgered by their partners to come, and often there is a considerable delay before they get around to booking the appointment. All this delay means the melanoma will likely be more advanced at the time of presentation, which usually means it will be more likely to metastasize (spread around the body).

The commonest site for melanoma in men is on the trunk (chest or back) and for women it's the legs. This is probably explained by the fact that in hot weather men often take off their shirts and women will wear skirts exposing their legs.

We are not surprised that there are more cases of melanoma diagnosed in Australia (7,850 cases) than in the UK (5,990 cases) each year (despite the UK having double the population of Australia). However, you may be dismayed to hear that more people die from melanoma in the UK than in Australia, 1600 deaths/year in the UK compared to 1000 in Australia. So why do more people die from melanoma in the UK than in Australia? There appears to be a number of factors compounding the problem in the UK, including our lack of sun protection awareness, an under estimation of the strength of the sun and our late presentation to the GP or dermatologist.

One of the most famous and most successful sun awareness campaigns globally was conceived in Australia more than 20 years ago. It used the slogan 'slip, slap, slop' which has become well know all over the world, and translates into slip on a shirt, slap on a hat and slop on some sunscreen. So, Australians are consequently much more aware of protecting themselves from the sun than perhaps we are in the UK.

So it does appear that we are at risk of melanoma when living in temperate climates and also slightly more likely to die from it. Do these figures for melanoma just reflect the fact that many of us have fair skin, or is it that we generally have sun-seeking behaviour and/or travel abroad to sunny climates? A combination of these factors is likely to play a role in the development of melanoma.

In 2015 Tishelman and colleagues conducted a study in four countries in Northern Europe (Norway/Sweden/Denmark/Northern Ireland) where they asked >8000 adults about awareness of risk factors for melanoma. Encouragingly, 91% recognised 'sunbed use' and 97% 'change in a mole', but only 63% recognised 'sunburn in childhood' as a risk factor. So, our awareness is improving but we need to do more to ensure the message is getting out there. We particularly need to protect children and young people as they have thinner, more vulnerable skin.

It is estimated that 25% of sun exposure occurs before the age of 18 years. The latest research suggests that melanoma and basal cell carcinomas are more closely linked to intermittent high intensity ultraviolet exposure (particularly in childhood and adolescence) whereas squamous cell carcinoma is more commonly associated with continuous or cumulative sun exposure over many years. It is estimated that 70-90% of melanomas result from exposure to strong sunlight. Squamous cell carcinoma can lead to a cancer on the lip, which seems to be linked to a lifetime of strong sun exposure, and smoking.

What are the reasons for the doubling of the number of cases of melanoma in the last 10 years? The appeal of tanning has been a relatively new phenomenon over the past 40 years. In the UK in Victorian times, being tanned was associated with manual labour outside in the fields and the wealthy prided themselves on not becoming tanned. Nowadays we associate tanning with holidays, travel abroad and looking 'healthy'. With cheaper air fares and more leisure time we are more likely to visit sunny destinations, leading to intermittent high intensity sun exposure, which is known to be associated with melanoma, particularly in the young.

Apart from fair skin and the sun, there is evidence that genetic predisposition to skin cancer may also play a role in the development of the disease. Some families have susceptibility to multiple dysplastic naevi (lots of atypical strange looking moles) and these families have a greater risk of melanoma. There is also a genetic link to disorders of DNA repair after sun damage, when abnormalities in the skin are not corrected and result in skin cancer.

Some melanomas however do occur on relatively sun-protected sites such as the bottom of the feet, palm of the hand, under the nails, at the back of the eye (retina) and in mucous membrane sites (rectum/vulva/oropharynx) so there must be other factors contributing to the risk here. Melanoma at these sites is equally common amongst all skin types whether fair or dark.

Basal cell carcinoma (BCC) is the most common skin cancer, they grow very slowly in the skin and they never spread around the body (metastasize) so many doctors consider them to be relatively harmless. They are most common on the face, particularly the 'mask' area where they often start as a small 'spot' and slowly over many months/years increases in size. If neglected or left BCC's increase in size, ulcerate and may destroy local structures.

When a doctor suspects a BCC is present they usually take a biopsy (sample) from the lesion under local anaesthetic so that the lesion can be examined histologically (down the microscope to look at the cells in detail). The reason for this is there are three main types of BCC, superficial (close to the skin surface), nodular (a 'ball of tumour' in the dermal skin layer) and infiltrative (finger-like projections of BCC spreading out through the skin). Depending on the subtype of BCC seen down the microscope then different treatment options will be considered.

Squamous cell carcinomas (SCC) is the second most common skin cancer in many countries including the UK. Its occurrence is thought to be related to chronic sun exposure and therefore is more common in those with fair sun-damaged skin. It can also appear in areas of skin that have been exposed to ionising radiation, arsenic, chronic wounds/ulcers/scars/burns, or arises from pre-cancerous lesions such as Bowen's disease and actinic keratosis (scaly bits of sun-damage on the skin). In people whose immune system is slightly lowered for whatever reason (patients who have had a transplant, HIV infection or lymphoma/leukaemia, or taking one of the newer biological therapies), they have an increased risk of developing an SCC.

Wart virus infections can also lead to increased risk for SCC. Other risk factors for SCC include smoking and working outside. SCC's usually start with a nodule (lump) on the skin which increases in size, is thickened on the top, may ulcerate and can be tender or painful. SCC's can metastasize and therefore are usually treated as soon as possible after the diagnosis has been made.

Skin Cancer Treatment

In the UK, most melanomas are excised on the same day that they are diagnosed by a dermatologist (the so-called 'see and treat' approach). Melanomas are initially cut out under local anaesthetic with a few millimetres margin of normal skin around them. The histopathologist then examines the melanoma down the microscope to determine how deep it goes down into the skin (the Breslow thickness): this depth then dictates the margin of the subsequent wide local excision (the scar is cut out and a little bit of extra skin around it).

The Breslow thickness is one of the most important factors in determining prognosis (outcome): in general the thicker the melanoma the poorer the prognosis. It is thought that most melanomas get deeper the longer they are allowed to grow in the skin, so early diagnosis and treatment increases the chances of survival, which for melanoma at five-years post-treatment is 92%.

Many skin cancers occur on the face (particularly BCC and SCC) and therefore skin surgery can be challenging to ensure vital structures (eyes, nose, mouth and ears) are preserved. The 'gold standard' for removing BCCs on the face is to make sure all the skin cancer has been removed whilst at the same time preserving as much normal skin around it as possible. This can be done directly by taking a few mms margin around the cancer or by a special technique called Mohs micrographic surgery.

In Mohs very thin layers of skin are taken from around the tumours and the margins are checked (the skin tissue removed is immediately cut up/stained and examined down the microscope) to ensure that all the tumour is out before the dermatology surgeon closes the defect (carries out a skilful reconstruction). Then the patient and the surgeon can feel confident that the BCC has been completely removed.

SCCs are usually treated under local anaesthetic by excising them (with a 5-10mm margin of normal skin around them), treating them with curettage and cautery (where they are scraped off and then cauterized three times; 'triple approach') or they can be treated by a non-surgical approach, namely radiotherapy.

Treatment of sun-damaged skin, such as pre-cancerous lesions (actinic keratosis, Bowen's disease, lentigo maligna) can be undertaken by 'freezing treatment' with liquid nitrogen (that has a temperature of minus 196 degrees Celsius), which kills the abnormal cells by freezing them. Pre-cancerous lesions or superficial BCCs can be 'scraped off' under local anaesthetic (curettage and cautery): the skin then heals up like a graze (no stitches needed) over a week or so.

Pre-cancerous lesions or superficial BCCs can also be treated with creams such as imiquimod (Aldara 5%) or Efudix (5-flourouricil). Aldara stimulates the immune cells (lymphocytes) to come into the skin where the cream is applied and then those cells start attacking the abnormal sun-damaged or cancerous cells locally. Efudix cream directly kills abnormal skin cells and leaves normal cells unharmed. Both creams will cause the skin to look red where they are applied and they usually need to be used for between six and 16 weeks to clear the lesions completely.

Photodynamic therapy (PDT) is another approach that can be used to treat pre-cancerous lesions and superficial BCCs. It is helpful to treat skin lesions that are very large and very thin. A photosensitizing cream (usually 5-aminolaevulinic acid ALA) is applied to the affected skin and covered with a plastic dressing for three to six hours, to enable the cream to penetrate. The excess cream is then removed and a special light is shone onto the skin for up to an hour. This can sting and burn a little during the treatment as the cancer cells that have taken up the ALA are killed by the light.

Radiotherapy can be used to treat primary SCCs and BCCs. The decision to opt for radiotherapy may be patient preference, or the site/size of the skin cancer may not be amenable for surgery. High energy X-rays are used to destroy the skin cancer cells and are delivered to the lesion in a number of treatment sessions over two to four weeks. The affected skin will become red and sore usually after the treatment had been completed, and will heal with a pale scar.

So there are lots of treatments for pre-skin cancer and skin cancer, and it is rarely fatal. So do seek advice from a medical practitioner if you are worried about any lesion on your skin. The earlier we treat melanoma the better. Prevention is definitely worthwhile by using high factor sunscreen on exposed vulnerable pale skin in strong sunlight. 'If in doubt check it out', and if we are in doubt about any lesion then we 'cut it out'.

Risk Factors for Developing Skin Cancer

- Naturally fair/light coloured skin.

- Skin that burns, freckles, turns red easily or becomes painful in the sun.

- A personal/family history of skin cancer.

- Blue or green eyes.

- Naturally blond or red/auburn hair.

- Exposure to the sun for many hours each day, during work/leisure.

- Sunburns, especially early in life.

- Using sun beds.

- Large number of 'atypical' moles (moles that look irregular).

- Smoking cigarettes (increased risk of squamous cell carcinoma).

- Longstanding (for months/years) non-healing wound/ulcer.

Self-Skin Checks:
What to look out for that might indicate melanoma

- The sudden appearance of a new irregular mole, or sudden irregular growth of a pre-existing mole.

- A mole that looks different from your other moles, that 'stands out from the crowd', the so-called 'ugly duckling sign'.

- A mole that spontaneously (without trauma) starts crusting, bleeding or oozing.

- A mole that seems to be moving off/growing more in one direction or another.

- A change in colour in a mole, so there are several colours within it.

When trying to assess any individual mole, the following simple checklist can be very helpful.

The ABCDE checklist:

- **A for asymmetrical** – melanomas often have two different 'halves' and an irregular shape.

- **B for border** – unlike most harmless moles, melanomas usually have a notched or ragged border.

- **C for colour** – melanomas may be a mix of several colours.

- **D for diameter** – melanomas are usually larger than 6mm (¼inch) in diameter (shirt button size).

- **E for evolution** – a mole that changes over time (shape/colour/size) can be a sign of melanoma.

What to look out for that might indicate basal cell carcinoma

- A lesion (usually on the face) that is slow growing over months/years and usually flesh coloured/slightly red.

- A bump/lump on the skin that feels firm to the touch (it has substance to it under the skin surface).

- Lesions that slowly and progressively increase in size and gradually crust or ulcerate.

- A lesion that never heals up, repeated crusting.

- Lesions that looks slightly shiny with a raised pearly-looking edge and may have prominent blood vessels in it.

- Something on the torso/limbs that looks like a patch of dry red skin that is not itchy and doesn't resolve with creams.

- A longstanding ulcerated area of skin that doesn't heal up as expected.

What to look out for that might indicate squamous cell carcinoma

- A rapidly growing (weeks/months) flesh-coloured nodule (lump) on the skin (usually at a sun-exposed site).

- The nodule may be quite firm underneath and quite thickened and scaly on the top.

- Lesions may be tender or painful and can crust, ulcerate, bleed and weep fluid.

- The nodule may be quite friable (breaks easily) if knocked or rubbed.

- Non-healing long-standing wound or ulcer with a raised/irregular edge.

Skin symptoms/signs that are unlikely to be skin cancer

- A skin lesion or mole that is just itchy.

- Something on the skin that is coming and going, rather than persistent and progressive.

- A dry warty brownish/tan coloured lesion that appears to be 'stuck onto the skin surface' (seborrheic keratosis, a harmless warty thickening of the top layer of the skin, often multiple).

- A static firm pea-sized circular lesion on the leg, occasionally itchy and has a brown ring around it (dermatofibroma, harmless scar-like lesion in the skin, may emanate from an old insect bite).

- Multiple lesions on the skin all appearing to be the same (skin tags, warty lesions, freckles).

Top tips for avoiding skin cancer

- Don't use sunbeds.

- Use high factor sunscreen (factor 50) on exposed fair skin, especially in children.

- Avoid sunburn by applying sunscreen before going out into the sun, and reapply.

What should you do if you are worried about your moles/skin cancer?

- Ask your general practitioner to have a look.

- Ask a dermatologist to have a look.

- If possible, ensure the doctor examines all your moles/skin at the consultation.

CHAPTER 13

DIY Skin Treatments

How to treat Sunburn.

Too much intense sun on a fair skin can lead to a sunburn. This is thankfully a rare occurrence for most of us, but it can be very severe when it happens and can make us feel quite unwell for 24 hours. Sunburn usually results from unexpectedly strong sun, such as when the air feels cold but the sun is intense, or when you fall asleep in the sun, or if there is a lot of reflection whilst out on the water. The first signs are usually the exposed skin looking red and feeling hot to the touch.

Cooling. As soon as you realise you have a sunburn, then try to **get your skin out of the sun** as soon as possible by going indoors, covering your skin with clothing and/or sitting in deep shade. You need to try to cool the burnt skin down as rapidly as possible. **Apply cold wet flannels** to the affected areas, or even ice wrapped in cloth if possible. Keep the **cold compress** applied to the affected skin for at least 15 minutes if possible. You know when you have done enough as when you take the cold compress away the skin no longer feels as if its burning. If as you take the compress away and the burning sensation recurs, then apply the cold cloth for a little longer.

Ibuprofen. If there are no contraindications (allergy, stomach ulceration) then adults should take Ibuprofen 400mg (check the dose on the packet/bottle for a child). The ibuprofen will help to reduce pain and swelling in the skin and should be taken regularly for the first 24 hours. Taking ibuprofen after food helps to reduce the chance of stomach irritation.

Moisturising Cream. Any soothing cooling cream (moisturiser, emollient, body lotion, Vaseline, 'Aftersun') can be applied to the affected skin (**keep the cream in the fridge** so it feels even more cooling when applied). Cream can be **applied every hour** if necessary, the more the better.

Blisters. If there are large tense blisters, then it is a good idea to **pop them using a sterile needle**. Pass a needle briefly into a flame to sterilise it, allow it to cool before puncturing the blisters. Puncture blisters near their base and press gently on the top of them to encourage the fluid to seep out into a piece of clean tissue paper. Keep the blister roof intact if possible.

Steroid Ointment. If you have a tube of steroid cream at home in the cupboard, then this can be applied to the sun burnt skin areas for the first few days. Some steroid creams can be bought over the counter at the chemist without a prescription (as they are quite mild). So if you don't have any already then try to buy **hydrocortisone ointment**/cream (any %) or the slightly stronger

Eumovate ointment/cream (clobetasone butyrate 0.05%), and apply this twice daily until the redness goes down (may take a few days).

Sometimes after an extensive severe sunburn you can actually feel sick and shivery. If that is the case then you need to **drink lots of water, and lie down in bed**. You will usually recover by the next day.

How to treat a burn to the skin from the cooker/oven/hot drink/firework/fire etc.

Cooling. As soon as you burn your skin on something very hot you need to cool the area down as rapidly as possible. **Ideally put the burnt area of skin under cold running water immediately**. Any delay in cooling can cause the effects of the burn to be much worse. If you get the affected skin under a cold running tap straight away, you can usually prevent blistering and ultimately pain.

The key however is to keep the skin under the cold running tap – for much longer than you think will be necessary. You will need to keep the affected skin under the cold running water for about 5-10 minutes (continuously). If you don't have cold water to hand you could use cold milk, or a soft drink or even beer. If you have **ice or a bag of frozen food** to hand, then this can be applied to the affected skin area instead of using cold running water. When you think you have applied the cold to the area for long enough, take it off and see if the burning sensation comes back, if it does then you need to apply the cold for longer.

If it is a baby or young child that gets burnt (such as a hot drink getting accidentally tipped over them), then you may need to **get the child into the sink/bath** and hold them so the affected skin is under the cold running water. They obviously won't like it, but ultimately if you can do this the result of the burn will be less harmful/severe and less likely to leave a scar afterwards.

Plastic covering. Burns can be covered with **clingfilm** or a clean **plastic bag**. This is especially helpful if any blisters appear in the burnt skin. The blisters can be carefully popped/punctured using a sterile needle (see explanation above). If it is a finger/hand that is burnt/blistering, then after the cold water/ice treatment apply Vaseline to the affected areas and put a plastic bag/Clingfilm over the affected hand to keep the ointment on and keep the air off it for 24 hours.

Steroid ointment (as above under Sunburn) can be applied to the burnt area twice a day for 24-48 hours to help reduce the inflammation in the affected skin.

If the burn is very extensive/severe and/or is affecting a baby/child – then I would suggest after you have completed the 'first aid' part of the treatment - cold water/ice and given them ibuprofen, that they may also require medical attention. You may need to take them to an Accident and Emergency Department or Minor Injuries Unit for expert help/advice and further treatment.

How to treat insect bite skin reactions

Insect bites are usually very itchy and it is almost impossible not to scratch them. They are often multiple and are usually on exposed skin. Insects frequently bite at dusk or at night, so you may wake up in the morning and suddenly feel multiple itchy bites particularly on your legs/ankles/arms.

Antihistamine. To try to reduce the itching take an **antihistamine tablet/liquid** regularly for the first 24-48 hours, you can buy these over the counter at the chemist. This help to reduce the reaction to the bites (which in fact is your immune cells reacting to the insect's saliva/proteins). Histamine release triggers itching, so antihistamines help to reduce further histamine release, and therefore reduce itch.

Steroid ointment plus plaster. Get a steroid ointment/cream (see above) and apply this twice daily to each bite and then cover the bites with a plaster (blister plasters are good for this – as they tend to stay on very well – you can cut them in half/quarters and apply the steroid underneath). The reason for the plaster is two-fold, this helps to drive the steroid ointment into the skin and also helps to protect the skin from scratching (which does tend to make the bite reactions worse).

Ice. If there is marked swelling with the bites (such as often occurs around the ankles), then it is worth applying ice to the area and elevating the leg/limb if possible. This will help to reduce the swelling and itching.

How to treat nettle rash/hives/wheals/urticaria

These types of rashes are bumpy and itchy and can be quite widespread. Obviously if you have sustained a nettle sting then it could be isolated to a small area of skin that touched the nettles, however hives/ wheals/ urticaria can be very widespread all over.

Nettle rash – is the reaction of the skin to a ground plant called the Stinging nettle (Urtica dioica). The leaves are covered in multiple tiny hairs (trichomes – which are like lots of tiny hollow needles). The hairs pierce our skin when we brush against the plant causing chemicals from the plants to enter our skin causing an irritant stinging sensation. The chemicals include histamine, serotonin and leukotrienes. The rash quickly becomes bumpy and painful.

Dock leaf. For hundreds of years, people have known that rubbing a dock-leaf (and in some countries a **plantain leaf**) on the affected nettle sting area of skin can reduce the rash and the stinging sensation, but how does this really help?

Well, in my personal experience it does seem to help, but I couldn't find any published scientific evidence to back this up. Some papers seem to quote research saying that dock-leaves contain a natural anti-histamine called chlorphenamine (which is present in the over the counter antihistamine Piriton). But the original paper they are referring to doesn't actually mention this, so at present there is no definite science behind the claim. Nonetheless it does seem to be soothing, but this just might be a mechanical effect in terms of rubbing off the micro hairs, or help to distract us from the stinging.

Antihistamine liquid or cream can be applied to the affected area.

Steroid ointment applied twice daily can also reduce the skin reaction.

Hives/wheals/urticaria

These types of rashes are usually very itchy and the rash is bumpy and flesh coloured or slightly red. The rash classically moves around so if you draw a circle around a particular bump with a pen, then within minutes or hours it will have gone down there, but may have moved elsewhere. These rashes can be caused by allergies to medications such as ibuprofen, codeine and antibiotics, but can also be triggered by infections, viral/bacterial or the cause may not be clear. This type of rash results from mast cells in our skin releasing their granules which include histamines and other chemicals. These chemicals trigger swelling of the skin and itching.

Antihistamines help to reduce the itching and swelling of urticaria, they start to take effect within about 20 minutes of taking them and should help the rash to resolve. Occasionally these types of rashes can come and go over days, weeks, months or even years and so antihistamines may need to be taken regularly to keep the rash controlled. The best antihistamines to take are the non-sedating ones that can be purchased over the counter at the chemist. If, however, these don't settle the rash down then it would be worth seeing your family doctor to see if you need stronger prescription antihistamines instead.

Sometimes these types of rashes can be accompanied by very marked swelling of the skin/lips/eyes and this is called angioedema. It is not usually harmful but can look very alarming. Antihistamines should help to get this swelling down.

If, however the swelling/angiooedema is inside the mouth/throat and the affected person is having difficulty breathing they should go straight to the emergency department and get immediate medical attention.

How to treat Head lice/nits

Head lice are very common indeed. Most children and indeed adults will have head lice at some point in their lives, but the good news is, they are easy to treat. Head lice are blood-sucking parasites, they prefer the dark so they tend to hang out at the back of the scalp and behind the ears, close to the skin. Head lice are passed from one person to another. Children, who are frequently in close proximity to each other, tend to pass them on more easily than adults. Lice are about the size of a match head – so can be seen with the naked eye if you look closely. It's easier to inspect someone else than look at your own scalp. However, if you need to do your own detective work then put your head over the bath or a sink and comb/brush vigorously and you will see any lice/nits as they fall out (if they are present). If you're inspecting someone else's scalp, then look closely at the hair behind the ears and at the back of the scalp for signs of lice and nits.

Anti-head lice treatment. The most effective treatment is to put a form of silicone oil (**dimeticone,** which can be bought over the counter at the chemist) onto dry hair (similar to the silicone that is found in hair conditioners) and then dry the hair with a hair dryer. Leave this on overnight (put an old towel on the pillow). The dried silicone solution kind of 'shrink wraps' the lice and suffocates them. Dimeticone, and indeed any chemical lice treatment only kills the lice and not the eggs, and therefore the treatment needs to be repeated after 7 days. This will ensure any eggs that have hatched after the first treatment and produced small lice (called nymphs) will now be killed by the second treatment.

Other chemical treatments include **permethrin and malathion** – which should also be applied to dry hair, left on overnight and then washed out in the morning. These applications should also be repeated after 7 days. There is increasing evidence that some head lice have become resistant to these chemicals, hence my current recommendation is the dimeticone where there is no documented resistance. Dimeticone is very cheap, non-toxic and easy to use (I have personal experience using it on myself, my husband and our 2 sons!)

Empty egg cases tend to look quite white, whereas the ones which are still alive tend to look almost translucent. Indeed, it can be hard to tell, so repeating the treatment after 7 days is best.

Physical lice/nit removal can be undertaken by combing, suction devices, etc. but this does require the affected person (usually a child) to sit still for repeated sessions of combing (either wet or dry) and in studies has been shown only to be effective if done very rigorously and repeatedly.

Chicken pox

Most of us will have chicken pox as a child. It's a relatively minor viral illness but the rash can be quite severe in some cases. The rash starts with a few small blisters that appear in crops and they then start to crust over. There are usually lots of blisters all at different stages of development. The blister fluid is contagious and chicken pox can be passed on by contact with this fluid, but more commonly it's transmitted by minute droplets sprayed into the air through breathing, coughing and sneezing. The incubation period (from when you get the infection to the first signs of the rash) is about 14 days.

There is no specific treatment for chicken pox, it's a mild viral illness that our immune system deals with and we recover after about 1 week. The rash itself can be uncomfortable and even itchy, and if this occurs then a soothing **antibacterial cream** (such as Dermol 500 cream) can be applied to help prevent cracking and secondary bacterial infection, whilst the skin is healing.

Steroid cream can also be applied to the spots once they have started to crust over, this reduces inflammation.

How to treat Molluscum contagiosum

This is a very common pox virus causing small round flesh coloured dimpled bumps to appear on the skin. They are often clustered in groups and are highly contagious (Molluscum contagiosum) – they are spread by touch. Although the virus is pretty harmless the multiple lesions can be unsightly and cause embarrassment. Having said that most kids will have them at some stage and they usually resolve spontaneously when the immune system starts to clear the virus. This can however take up to 2 years, as the virus is quite clever at evading the immune system cells. This is why some kids/adults would like to try some treatment to resolve the molluscum more quickly.

Hydrogen peroxide 1% cream can be bought over the counter and is a disinfectant cream. It has been shown to kill many types of bacteria and some fungi/viruses. When the hydrogen peroxide is applied to the individual molluscum lesions it isn't thought to be specifically killing the pox virus, it is more likely to be just causing irritation to the skin, and this in turn stimulates the immune system to send white cells (lymphocytes) into the area which start to 'mop-up' the virus. Avoid putting the cream anywhere on the face, just treat lesions elsewhere on the body twice daily. Once the lesions look inflamed and 'angry' (this may take a few weeks) then stop applying the hydrogen peroxide cream– just let the immune system do the rest. Once the immune system has 'recognised' the virus then all the molluscum lesions can clear up very rapidly over a few weeks. Once you are immune you are unlikely to get the molluscum back again.

There is a **5% hydrogen peroxide lotion** available, (Molludab) that can be prescribed by a healthcare provider if the 1% isn't helping.

Rarely doctors might treat a few molluscum (off the face) with **liquid nitrogen** (cryotherapy, a very cold spray), but the risk with this treatment is that this is more likely to leave a mark or scar on the skin once the molluscum has cleared, so this should be used only in very persistent cases. It's useful to bear in mind that if molluscum are left to clear naturally, they won't leave any scars or marks on the skin.

How to treat Cold sores

Sores on the lips caused by the herpes simples virus (HSV)– so called 'cold sores' are very common. They start with a kind of tingling sensation at the site, usually on the edge of the lip (but can occur on the chin/nose/elsewhere on the face) and then quickly form a small bump which develops into a small blister. This then 'pops' and the lesion becomes crusted. Cold sore virus is passed from one person to another through touch, and once someone has the virus (as do 90% of us) they have it for life. Between 'attacks' the virus sits in the nerve root and then can appear on the skin surface (usually at the same place each time) as a small blister again. Attacks can be triggered by the cold (as the name suggests), minor trauma (such as biting/knocking your lip/dental work), sunshine and if you are feeling 'run down' generally with a viral illness.

There are actually two types of herpes simplex virus causing cold sores, one mainly on the face – Type I, and one mainly in the genital area – Type II. The facial type is more common.

Aciclovir cream 5% should be applied to the cold sore skin as soon as you feel the 'attack' is coming on. If you feel a tingling or feel/see a small bump starting to appear apply the aciclovir cream every 4 hours. You can buy aciclovir cream over the counter at the chemist. The cream should be used for 5-10 days to clear the cold sore. Studies show the acyclovir cream helps to speed up healing by about 24-48 hours compared to placebo.

As the area starts to dry out the lip/skin can be vulnerable to cracking so apply plenty of **lipsalve and/or Vaseline** to the affected area to try to prevent painful cracking.

If you have very severe/frequent attacks of cold sores around your mouth or on your genital skin, then your family doctor may prescribe aciclovir tablets to take for a few days. The tablets have to be taken within the first 72 hours of the attack starting for them to be of any help. I sometimes give patients a prescription to get a supply of aciclovir tablets so they have them at home ready for any subsequent outbreaks.

How to treat dry cracked lips/corners of mouth

Dry cracked lips are very common particularly when the weather is cold and wet. Also, if you have a blocked nose and tend to 'mouth breathe' then the lips can also become quite dry, 'chapped' and feel sore. Lips can even crack/ bleed and this can be painful when trying to eat/drink. Because the lips feel dry there is a tendency to lick them (often done subconsciously) and this makes the problem much worse. Saliva contains enzymes and chemicals which irritate the already dry and inflamed lips, and this results in a vicious cycle, which can be hard to break.

Applying regular **Vaseline and/or lipsalve/lip balm** literally every hour is very effective at helping to heal the lips. This will also reduce the tendency to lick the lips and if you do, then the lips will be protected by a film of Vaseline. If protective Vaseline/lipsalve is applied very regularly then the condition will get better within a few days to a week.

If you ask your pharmacist you may also be able to buy over the counter **lipsalve containing 1% hydrocortisone** (CortiBalm, FixMySkin) this will help to reduce inflammation at the same time as moisturising the lips and will promote healing. This is especially useful to be applied just before going to sleep.

How to treat Corns/hard skin on feet/toes

Where our shoes press on our feet/toes the skin naturally becomes slightly thicker as a protective mechanism. However, if the skin becomes very thickened at a particular skin site, then it can become painful when shoes press on it (hard corn).

This is very common and can usually be managed quite easily by ensuring footwear isn't too tight and that the thickened areas of skin are **rubbed down on a regular basis** to prevent them becoming too thick. Rubbing the skin down is best after a bath or shower when the skin is slightly softer.

Acne

It's tough when you suffer from acne spots, so as parents we need to try to ensure that we are as supportive as possible when our kids get acne. It's best not to say things like 'you'll grow out of it' or 'no one will notice'. It can really affect confidence and self-esteem, so early intervention is usually appreciated by sufferers. Firstly, buy some of the **acne prone skin face washes** from the chemist, this help to remove excess oil from the skin surface and unblock the pores which get clogged in acne. Then buy a topical cream over the counter such as one containing **benzoyl peroxide (4-5%)**. This is really quite effective if used every night onto the active spots. It is anti-inflammatory and will help unblock the glands with its mild peeling effect. The other over the counter preparation you could try is **nicotinamide gel** which can be applied twice daily to inflamed red acne spots. Acne can be disguised with make-up/camouflage cream (try Dermablend) and this won't make the acne worse. A little bit of sunshine and salt water can also help. If these simple measures really aren't helping sufficiently then do make an appointment to see your local doctor to get some prescription treatment. Much better to treat acne early and thoroughly than try to deal with scars later. Tablet options include antibiotics (should be taken for a minimum of 3-6 months), for females some types of oral contraceptive pills. Ultimately for more severe or refractory acne, oral isotretinoin (which is a type of vitamin A derivative), this is usually only prescribed by dermatologists.

Warts

Are very common, about 90% of us will get a wart at some point in our lives. They are caused by the human papilloma virus (HPV) and produce rough thickenings of the skin, often on the fingers and soles of the feet, but any skin site can be affected. HPV is passed from one person to another. Also, if you touch your own warts and then touch another part of your skin, you can also spread them (auto-inoculation). Warts on the soles of the feet (verrucas) are often acquired through walking bare-foot on communal floors such as changing rooms at the swimming pool/gym/family bathroom where HPV can sit in wait. When the skin is wet, it is more vulnerable to HPV and it tends to get implanted at weight-bearing skin sites on the feet. A top tip for avoiding verrucas would be to wear **flip flops/beach shoes** etc. in communal showers/changing rooms.

HPV is quite a clever virus as it sits in the very top layer of the skin, and isn't noticed by our immune cells. Because of this the wart can be present for months/years without any kind of reaction from our bodies to it. All the treatments used to help get rid of warts try to physically remove the wart infected skin by **rubbing it/filing it/paring it down** and then irritating the remaining wart underneath – usually by applying **salicylic acid in plasters/liquids. This should be repeated every day**. Ideally the wart should be **covered with a plaster** to help drive the salicylic acid into the wart and prevent further viral spread. You can buy Pickles Ointment (50% salicylic acid) online, which applied daily to warts on the feet/hands can be highly effective. About 80% of warts will clear if they are treated daily with rubbing down, high percentage salicylic acid and a plaster to cover.

Some studies advocate the use of **duct tape** that can be bought from the DIY shop. This can be cut to size, placed over the warts and changed every 2-3 days. It is thought something in the glue of the tape helps to kill the HPV. Some studies have shown better results than others, so more studies are underway to see how much it helps.

Freezing cold spray can also be used to treat warts and you can buy a form of this over the counter at the chemist. The warts should always be rubbed down first before the cold spray is applied, as this helps the spray to penetrate into the wart and make the treatment more effective. Multiple freezing treatment episodes are usually needed to clear the warts. Over the counter cold sprays tend to be less effective than liquid nitrogen (cryotherapy) as the former are around -60 degrees and the latter -190 degrees centigrade.

Skin infections – pustules/boil/carbuncle/impetigo

Bacterial skin infections are really very common. Most of us will get an infected 'spot' at some point. Bacteria get into our skin quite easily, especially if the skin is broken, damaged or inflamed. Initially the skin may feel tender or painful to touch and you may see redness and swelling. A pustule (cloudy liquid) may form at the site and you may see some golden coloured crusting. These are all signs and symptoms of bacterial skin infections.

Wash infected skin with an **antiseptic wash**, you can use salt-water (Epsom salts), dilute chlorhexidine or iodine. Remove any crust/crud from them skin surface. Repeat twice a day.

For pustules/boils/abscesses you can apply a **warm clean flannel (moist heat)** to the affected skin area, this helps to dilate blood vessels and bring inflammatory cells and pus to the surface. Once pus is at the surface it can drain, which relives pressure and pain and the healing process can start. Don't be tempted to squeeze the skin around the boil as this can cause the pus to go down into the deep skin and may lead to scarring. Obviously if the boil or abscess is very large you may need to attend your local doctors or minor injuries department to have the lesion **incised and drained** under local anaesthetic. Your doctor may also want to prescribe a short course of oral antibiotics. If you develop recurrent boils and other members of your household are similarly affected your doctor may take swabs and ask the laboratory to see if the bacteria contain **PVL toxin/or MRSA**, which may require a **decolonisation treatment** (an antibacterial wash plus antibiotic up the nose for a few days) as well as oral antibiotics for a few weeks.

Jellyfish sting

Luckily jellyfish stings are uncommon and usually only occur whilst swimming in the sea. Dead jellyfish washed up on the beach can still give a nasty sting if their tentacles are touched. There is some medical evidence to support **washing the sting site with salt water** rather than freshwater afterwards. Hot/warm water (as warm as can be tolerated) **for 30-60 minutes**, (be careful not to burn the skin) is more effective at relieving pain and swelling than cold water. Hot sea water may be difficult to access at the beach – but nonetheless warm salty water is more effective than cold fresh water. **Remove any tentacles** or stinging cells with a clean stick or shell. The pain should start to ease off after 20 minutes. **Painkillers** such as paracetamol and Ibuprofen can help each the pain and swelling. If the skin is still red the following day, then apply **steroid cream** to the area (such as hydrocortisone or Eumovate).

The use of vinegar to wash off stinging tentacles is controversial. There is evidence vinegar reduces the number of nematocysts (small poisonous sacs) that discharge venom, however those already 'fired' release more venom when in contact with vinegar, leading increased pain. No one advises the use of urine to wash the sting either (there is no evidence it helps, and it may add insult to injury). NHS Cornwall is recommending using shaving foam to jelly fish sting sites (but it is doubtful many beach-goers will have this with them, and I am unsure what the evidence for this is).

Splinters

These are small slivers of wood/plant material/metal that get into the skin through minor scrapes and can be quite painful. **Wash the affected area** of skin before attempting to remove the splinter with **clean tweezers**. It can be helpful to use a magnifying glass or at least good lighting to help you locate and remove the splinter from the skin. Sometimes it might be necessary to break the skin over the top of the splinter, use a **sterile needle** or pin to do this. (you can use alcohol hand rub to clean the needle and the tweezers). If the splinters are very fragile such as from fibreglass or plant bristles, then using **duct/electrical tape**. Press the tape firmly onto the skin and then carefully lift off, repeat if necessary to remove all the splinters. Once the splinter is out, clean the skin thoroughly and apply a plaster. Ensure you are vaccinated against tetanus every 10 years.

Stings wasp/bee

First thing to do is immediately **remove the stinger**, you can use a debit card, coin or cloth (to knock/scrape it off). **Wash** the skin with soap and water and **apply ice/frozen peas** to reduce pain and swelling. **Antihistamines** and cold numbing spray (anaesthetic) can give relief; as can **painkillers** such as paracetamol and ibuprofen. Avoid squeezing the skin, using vinegar or bicarbonate of soda which may make things worse. Any signs of a severe allergic reactions to the sting can be serious so ensure the person gets to hospital as soon as possible.

Blisters

Painful clear fluid filled swellings (blisters) on the skin can result from numerous different causes. The most common are burns, friction, trauma, bites and skin infections/allergies. Whatever the cause the immediate treatment is the same. **Wash the skin** with soap and water, **puncture the blister** close to its base with a sterile needle (can be cleaned with alcohol hand gel, or passed through a flame and cooled). **Gently press down** on the blister with a clean tissue and the liquid will come out. Try to **keep the roof on the blister** as this will help to reduce the level of pain and protect the underlying raw skin from infection. Cover with plain **Vaseline and a plaster** (blister platers can be very helpful for protecting the skin and helping to reduce pain).

Graze/abrasion/friction burn

Wash the skin with soap and water. Apply **Vaseline** or any oily cream to the skin and cover with a **plaster**.

Topical **steroid ointment** can be helpful if the surrounding skin gets very red.

Cat/dog/human bites

Bites can be quite nasty as sharp teeth make very small deep puncture wounds in the skin and the saliva from the animal/human is full of germs (mainly bacteria) from the mouth. **Wash the skin** thoroughly and **allow some bleeding** as this helps to wash away bacteria. Apply a piece of **clean tissue** and press on the area whilst **elevating** it. Once the bleeding has stopped clean again with **soap and water**. Apply **antiseptic ointment** generously to the wound and cover with a **plaster**. Painkillers can be helpful. If the bite is severe and affecting the face or fingers/hand then you may need to seek medical attention to check for damage to deep structures under the skin (tendons, nerves). You may need a **tetanus** vaccination (booster every 10 years) and possibly **oral antibiotics**.

Mouth ulcers

These are really common and usually last only a few days, but they can be very painful and affect eating/drinking. It's not clear what causes mouth ulcers but we do know that minor trauma in the mouth can cause them, acid fruits, poorly fitting braces/dentures and they are more likely to occur if we are 'under the weather' with a cough/cold/viral illness. At the chemist, you can buy an **antibacterial mouthwash**, **painkilling gel/spray** with anaesthetic in it to numb the pain and also **corticosteroid lozenges** (for those over the age of

12 years). If ulcers persist for more than 3 weeks, then it would be a good idea to see your local doctor of dentist.

Halitosis

Bad breath is caused by gram-negative anaerobic bacteria in the mouth. We all have a bit of that when we wake up in the morning, and it's **easily removed by brushing our teeth and tongue** with toothpaste. If you have gum disease, holes in your teeth (caries) or just poor dental hygiene, then halitosis can become more persistent throughout the day. **Daily tongue cleaning**, especially the back of the tongue can really help to get rid of the bacteria. **Mouthwash and toothpaste containing oxidants** can be particularly helpful at keeping the problem at bay. If the problem persists, see a dental hygienist to get help and advice.

Body odour/sweating

So-called body odour (bromhidrosis) comes from bacteria on the skin that break down sweat into fatty acids that have an unpleasant odour. There is some research that shows that some of us are less likely to be aware of the smell than others (the lining of our nostrils may not be able to detect certain odour molecules). The more we sweat the more bacteria are likely to be present and the greater the chance of odour.

To combat body odour, **wash the skin at least once a day** with soap and water, especially the armpits, groin and feet. Some people may need to bathe more than once a day. **Antibacterial washes** (containing chlorhexidine) to troublesome areas can be very helpful. **Antiperspirant** applied to the sites can help to reduce sweating and **deodorant** contains perfume to disguise the fatty acid smell. There are some stronger antiperspirant preparations that you can buy at the chemist containing **aluminium chloride hexahydrate**, these can be very effective although a little irritant to sensitive skin.

Sweaty/smelly feet – pitted keratolysis

This is a condition where the skin of the soles of the feet becomes peppered with tiny holes or pits, and the feet have a very strong unpleasant odour. This is caused by colonisation of the skin by bacteria called *Corynebacterium*. This is more likely to occur in people whose feet sweat profusely. The bacteria thrive in the warm moist environment and their enzymes dissolve the horny skin cells leading to pits. The bacteria produce sulphur which causes the bad smell.

The good news is this condition can be treated by **washing the feet twice daily in chlorhexidine** solution. Your local doctor can prescribe a **topical antibiotic cream** (fusidic acid or erythromycin) that can be applied to the affected areas. It is also helpful to **wear cotton socks**, well-ventilated shoes and use **antiperspirant on the feet** alternate days. Change the inner soles of your footwear to help prevent re-infection after treatment.

Athletes foot/jock itch

Superficial fungal infection of the skin is very common in adults and two of the most problematic areas are in between the toes and the groin area. These fungi prefer warm moist skin, so they thrive if the feet are hot and sweaty, hence the term 'athlete's foot'. Walking bearfoot in communal areas where the fungal spores persist for months can be the source of infection. The skin becomes itchy, dry and occasionally red or white.

Use **terbinafine 1% cream** (buy this at the chemist) twice daily (for 6-8 weeks) to the affected areas on the feet and in the groin. Consider investing in **new underwear, socks and shoes**, as reinfection with fungal spores in clothing can be a problem. **Dry the skin carefully** after bathing and consider applying an **anti-fungal talcum powder** to the worst affected areas for a few weeks. If athletes foot always seems to return, consider buying some 'toe-spacers' from the chemist to allow fresh air to circulate between your toes, which makes the skin environment less appealing to recurrent fungi.

1